FIBROMYALGIA
Understanding Symptoms, Treatments, and Self-Help Strategies

Megan Morris

Copyright © 2024 by Rivercat Books LLC

All rights reserved.

No portion of this book may be reproduced in any form without written permission from the publisher or author, except as permitted by U.S. copyright law.

CONTENTS

Introduction	1
Chapter 1: Fibromyalgia 101	4
Chapter 2: The Signs & Symptoms	15
Chapter 3: Getting Diagnosed	21
Chapter 4: Treating Fibromyalgia with Medication	30
Chapter 5: Additional Treatment Options	35
Chapter 6: Self-Help Techniques	54
Chapter 7: Supplements and Herbal Remedies	66
Chapter 8: Living with Fibromyalgia	71
Chapter 9: The Future of Fibromyalgia	82
Conclusion	86

INTRODUCTION

Living with fibromyalgia can feel like navigating through an uncharted territory filled with chronic pain, fatigue, and an array of perplexing symptoms. For many, the journey to understanding and managing fibromyalgia is fraught with confusion and frustration. Whether you are someone who has been diagnosed with fibromyalgia, believe you might have it and are seeking more information, or a loved one wanting to support someone with the condition, this book is here to guide you through this complex landscape.

Fibromyalgia: Understanding Symptoms, Treatments, and Self-Help Strategies is designed to be a comprehensive yet accessible resource for anyone affected by this condition. While it is not intended to replace medical advice, this book aims to provide valuable insights and practical strategies that can empower you to take control of your health and well-being.

Fibromyalgia is a condition that has often been misunderstood and misdiagnosed. In this book, we begin by delving into the history of fibromyalgia, tracing its recognition and understanding through the years. Chapter 1, Fibromyalgia 101, offers a foundational overview, explaining what fibromyalgia is and dispelling common myths and misconceptions.

Recognizing the signs and symptoms is a crucial step in seeking help and managing fibromyalgia. Chapter 2, The Signs & Symptoms, provides a detailed exploration of the common and less common symptoms that characterize this condition. From widespread pain and fatigue to cognitive difficulties and mood disturbances, understanding the full spectrum of symptoms can help you identify and address them more effectively.

Getting a proper diagnosis is often one of the most challenging aspects of fibromyalgia. Chapter 3, Getting Diagnosed, outlines the diagnostic process, explaining the criteria that must be met and the various tests and procedures involved. It also discusses the importance of ruling out similar conditions and provides guidance on who to consult for a diagnosis.

Treatment options for fibromyalgia are diverse, ranging from medications to alternative therapies. Chapter 4, Treating Fibromyalgia with Medication, discusses the different medications that are commonly prescribed, including how they work and their potential side effects. Chapter 5, Additional Treatment Options, explores other therapies such as physical therapy, myotherapy, chiropractic care, injections, and massage therapy, offering a holistic view of the available treatments.

In addition to medical treatments, self-help strategies play a vital role in managing fibromyalgia symptoms. Chapter 6, Self-Help Techniques, provides practical advice on diet, sleep, exercise, stress management, and maintaining a symptom tracking journal. These strategies can help you take an active role in managing your condition and improving your quality of life.

Supplements and herbal remedies can also provide relief for some individuals with fibromyalgia. Chapter 7, Supplements and Herbal Remedies, explores various natural therapies that may help alleviate symptoms and support overall health. From vitamins and minerals to herbal extracts, this chapter offers insights into alternative options for symptom management.

Living with fibromyalgia requires more than just medical treatment; it involves adapting your lifestyle and finding ways to thrive despite the challenges. Chapter 8, Living with Fibromyalgia, discusses strategies for minimizing the impact of fibromyalgia on work, school, home life, and social interactions. It offers practical tips for maintaining a good quality of life and finding balance in daily activities.

Finally, Chapter 9, The Future of Fibromyalgia, looks ahead to what the future holds for fibromyalgia research and treatment. With emerging therapies, ongoing studies, and growing awareness, there is hope for more effective management and better outcomes for those living with fibromyalgia.

Throughout this book, you will find information, guidance, and support to help you navigate the complexities of fibromyalgia. By understanding the condition and exploring various treatment and self-help strategies, you can take proactive steps to manage your symptoms and improve your quality of life. Whether you are newly diagnosed, have been living with fibromyalgia for years, or are supporting a loved one, this book is your companion on the journey to better health and well-being.

CHAPTER 1: FIBROMYALGIA 101

Fibromyalgia is a complex and often misunderstood condition characterized by widespread musculoskeletal pain, fatigue, and tenderness in localized areas. Unlike acute pain caused by injury or illness, fibromyalgia pain persists without an obvious cause, often fluctuating in intensity and location. This chronic condition affects the way the brain processes pain signals, amplifying the perception of pain throughout the body.

People with fibromyalgia may also experience a range of other symptoms, including sleep disturbances, cognitive difficulties (often referred to as "fibro fog"), and sensitivity to temperature, light, and sound. Despite the lack of a visible injury or inflammation, the pain and fatigue associated with fibromyalgia can be severe and debilitating, significantly impacting daily activities and quality of life.

Fibromyalgia is not a new condition, and its recognition as a legitimate medical diagnosis has evolved over time. Today, it is understood as a central sensitization disorder, meaning the nervous system becomes overly sensitive to stimuli that would not normally cause pain.

The History of Fibromyalgia

The history of fibromyalgia is a fascinating journey through centuries of medical literature, cultural observations, and evolving scientific understanding. While the term "fibromyalgia" is relatively modern, descriptions of symptoms that closely resemble those of fibromyalgia can be traced back to ancient civilizations.

In ancient Egypt, medical texts such as the Ebers Papyrus, dating back to 1550 BCE, describe conditions involving widespread pain and fatigue. These early records hint at the existence of fibromyalgia-like symptoms, though the understanding and context were vastly different from modern interpretations. Similarly, in ancient Greece, Hippocrates, often hailed as the father of medicine, documented cases of chronic musculoskeletal pain without an apparent cause. His observations laid the groundwork for recognizing the persistence of pain beyond immediate injury or illness.

As medical knowledge progressed through the Middle Ages and into the Renaissance, chronic pain conditions continued to be acknowledged, though they were often poorly understood and variously attributed to imbalances in bodily humors or spiritual maladies. The 17th century saw the term "muscular rheumatism" emerge in medical texts, an early attempt to categorize conditions characterized by widespread pain in muscles and joints. This term, while not entirely accurate, represented a significant step towards recognizing a distinct syndrome that we now understand as fibromyalgia.

The 19th century marked a turning point in the medical community's approach to chronic pain. Physicians began to observe and document cases of what they termed "neurasthenia" and "nervous exhaustion," conditions that bore striking similarities to modern descriptions of fibromyalgia. These conditions were often associated with the stresses of modern life and were predominantly diagnosed in women. This period also saw the beginnings of more systematic studies into chronic pain and fatigue syndromes.

In the early 20th century, the term "fibrositis" was coined, reflecting the belief that inflammation of the fibrous tissues and muscles caused chronic pain. This theory held sway for several decades and was influential in the medical community's approach to diagnosing and treating chronic pain conditions. However, as research methods improved, the absence of inflammatory markers in many patients led to the term falling out of favor. The need for a more accurate understanding of the condition became apparent.

The significant breakthrough came in 1976 when Dr. Philip Hench introduced the term "fibromyalgia," derived from "fibro" (fibrous tissues), "myo" (muscle), and "algia" (pain). This new terminology marked a departure from the outdated inflammation model and began to focus on the pain experience and its neurological underpinnings. The American College of Rheumatology's establishment of diagnostic criteria for fibromyalgia in 1990 was a milestone that significantly advanced the recognition and study of the condition. These criteria included widespread pain lasting more than three months and the presence of tender points in specific body areas. This formalization was crucial in legitimizing fibromyalgia as a distinct medical condition and paved the way for further research and understanding.

Throughout the late 20th and early 21st centuries, advances in neuroimaging and pain research revealed that fibromyalgia is likely a central sensitization disorder. This understanding posits that fibromyalgia involves changes in the central nervous system, leading to increased sensitivity to pain. These insights have shifted the focus of fibromyalgia research and treatment towards understanding how the brain and spinal cord process pain signals.

Cultural perceptions of fibromyalgia have also evolved significantly. Once dismissed by some as a psychological or "hysterical" condition, fibromyalgia is now recognized as a legitimate medical syndrome with complex physiological and neurological components. This shift has been driven by the tireless advocacy of patients, healthcare providers, and researchers dedicated to shedding light on this debilitating condition.

What Causes Fibromyalgia?

Despite extensive research, the exact cause of fibromyalgia remains elusive. It is widely accepted that fibromyalgia is a multifactorial condition, meaning it likely results from a combination of genetic, environmental, and psychological factors. Here are some leading theories on what might cause fibromyalgia:

Genetic Predisposition

The notion that fibromyalgia may have a genetic component is supported by a growing body of research. Studies have shown that fibromyalgia tends to run in families, suggesting that genetic factors may contribute to the condition's development. Researchers have identified specific genetic variations that might increase an individual's susceptibility to fibromyalgia. These variations are often found in genes involved in the regulation of pain perception and the stress response.

One of the primary areas of focus has been genes that influence the function of neurotransmitters, such as serotonin, norepinephrine, and dopamine. These chemicals play crucial roles in modulating pain signals in the brain and spinal cord. Variations in genes responsible for the production, release, and reuptake of these neurotransmitters can lead to abnormalities in pain processing. For example, certain polymorphisms in the serotonin transporter gene (5-HTT) have been associated with altered pain sensitivity and a higher risk of developing fibromyalgia.

Additionally, genes involved in the hypothalamic-pituitary-adrenal (HPA) axis, which regulates the body's stress response, have also been implicated. Dysregulation of the HPA axis can result in abnormal cortisol levels, a hormone that helps manage stress and inflammation. Abnormal cortisol responses are often observed in individuals with fibromyalgia, suggesting that genetic factors affecting the HPA axis may contribute to the condition's development.

Family studies provide further evidence of a genetic predisposition. First-degree relatives of individuals with fibromyalgia are significantly more likely to develop the condition compared to the general population. Twin studies have also shown higher concordance rates for fibromyalgia among monozygotic (identical) twins than dizygotic (fraternal) twins, reinforcing the role of genetic factors.

However, it is essential to understand that genetic predisposition alone does not determine whether someone will develop fibromyalgia. The condition is multifactorial, meaning that environmental factors, lifestyle choices, and psychological stressors interact with genetic susceptibility to influence its onset and progression. For instance, a person with a genetic predisposition may not develop fibromyalgia unless they encounter significant physical or emotional stressors that trigger the condition.

Central Sensitization

Central sensitization is a key concept in understanding the pathology of fibromyalgia. It refers to the process by which the central nervous system, including the brain and spinal cord, becomes hypersensitive to pain stimuli. In individuals with fibromyalgia, this heightened sensitivity leads to an exaggerated perception of pain, even in response to stimuli that are not typically painful.

At the core of central sensitization is the phenomenon of neuroplasticity, where the nervous system adapts and changes in response to repeated stimuli. In the context of fibromyalgia, this adaptation is maladaptive, resulting in the amplification of pain signals. Normally, pain signals are modulated by the brain and spinal cord to prevent an overreaction to minor injuries or irritations. However, in fibromyalgia, this modulation process is disrupted.

Several mechanisms contribute to central sensitization. One significant factor is the persistent activation of pain pathways. When pain signals are continuously sent to the brain, the neurons involved in transmitting these signals become more responsive over time. This increased responsiveness, or hyperexcitability, means that even normal sensory inputs can be perceived as painful. Additionally, changes in the levels of neurotransmitters such as glutamate and substance P, which facilitate the transmission of pain signals, further enhance this sensitivity.

Functional and structural changes in the brain also play a critical role. Neuroimaging studies have shown that individuals with fibromyalgia exhibit increased activity in pain-processing areas of the brain, such as the insula and the anterior cingulate cortex. These regions are involved in the emotional and cognitive aspects of pain perception. Moreover, there is evidence of reduced gray matter volume in areas of the brain responsible for inhibiting pain, suggesting a diminished capacity to regulate pain signals effectively.

Another contributing factor to central sensitization is the dysfunction of the descending inhibitory pain pathways. These pathways normally act to suppress pain signals at the level of the spinal cord, preventing them from reaching the brain. In fibromyalgia, this inhibitory system is often impaired, allowing more pain signals to pass through and be perceived by the brain.

Genetic predispositions may also influence the development of central sensitization. Variations in genes involved in neurotransmitter systems and pain regulation can affect an individual's susceptibility to heightened pain sensitivity. This genetic component, combined with environmental and psychological stressors, can trigger and sustain central sensitization.

The concept of central sensitization helps explain why fibromyalgia patients often experience widespread pain and sensitivity to non-painful stimuli, such as light touch or mild pressure. It also accounts for the common comorbid symptoms of fibromyalgia, including fatigue, sleep disturbances, and cognitive difficulties.

These symptoms are believed to result from the same underlying neural mechanisms that amplify pain signals.

Physical and Emotional Trauma

Physical and emotional trauma are significant factors in the development and exacerbation of fibromyalgia, offering a compelling explanation for the onset of symptoms in many individuals. Trauma, whether physical or emotional, can act as a powerful trigger for the condition, setting off a cascade of changes in the nervous system that lead to the persistent pain and sensitivity characteristic of fibromyalgia.

Physical trauma refers to any injury or bodily harm that impacts the body. This can include events such as car accidents, surgeries, or severe physical injuries. For many people, fibromyalgia symptoms appear or worsen following such traumatic events. The link between physical trauma and fibromyalgia is believed to be related to the body's stress response. When the body experiences a traumatic injury, it activates the hypothalamic-pituitary-adrenal (HPA) axis, resulting in the release of stress hormones like cortisol. While this response is crucial for immediate survival and recovery, prolonged activation can lead to changes in pain processing pathways, making the nervous system more sensitive to pain signals. This phenomenon, known as central sensitization, means that pain from an injury may persist long after the physical damage has healed, and even non-painful stimuli can become painful.

Emotional trauma, which encompasses a wide range of experiences including childhood abuse, domestic violence, significant loss, and other severe psychological stressors, also plays a critical role in the onset of fibromyalgia. Emotional trauma can lead to chronic stress, which has profound effects on the body and brain. Chronic stress alters the functioning of the HPA axis and the autonomic nervous system, both of which are involved in the regulation of pain and stress responses. Prolonged exposure to stress hormones can enhance the sensitivity of pain pathways, contributing to the development of fibromyalgia.

Research has shown that individuals with a history of emotional trauma are more likely to develop fibromyalgia. This connection is supported by studies that have found higher rates of adverse childhood experiences among fibromyalgia patients compared to the general population. Emotional trauma can leave lasting imprints on the brain, particularly in regions involved in emotion regulation and pain perception, such as the amygdala and prefrontal cortex. These changes can predispose individuals to heightened pain sensitivity and difficulty managing stress, both hallmarks of fibromyalgia.

Neurochemical Imbalances

Neurochemical imbalances are a significant factor in the pathophysiology of fibromyalgia, influencing both the perception of pain and the regulation of mood and sleep. The brain and nervous system rely on a delicate balance of neurotransmitters—chemical messengers that transmit signals between nerve cells—to function properly. In individuals with fibromyalgia, this balance is often disrupted, leading to an array of symptoms.

One of the key neurotransmitters involved in fibromyalgia is serotonin. Serotonin plays a crucial role in regulating pain, mood, and sleep. Research has shown that individuals with fibromyalgia often have lower levels of serotonin in the brain. This deficiency can lead to heightened pain sensitivity, as serotonin is involved in the inhibition of pain pathways. Moreover, low serotonin levels are associated with mood disorders such as depression and anxiety, which are common comorbidities in fibromyalgia patients. This connection helps explain why many fibromyalgia patients experience both chronic pain and mood disturbances.

Another important neurotransmitter is norepinephrine, which is involved in the body's stress response and helps regulate pain and mood. Like serotonin, norepinephrine levels are often found to be altered in fibromyalgia patients. Low levels of norepinephrine can result in an inadequate stress response, contributing to the persistent fatigue and increased pain sensitivity observed in fibromyalgia. This imbalance can also affect concentration and cognitive function, exacerbating the "fibro fog" that many patients report.

Dopamine, another critical neurotransmitter, also plays a role in fibromyalgia. Dopamine is essential for regulating mood, motivation, and the brain's reward system. Disruptions in dopamine levels can lead to reduced pain tolerance and increased sensitivity to pain. This imbalance may also contribute to the high prevalence of mood disorders in fibromyalgia patients. Studies have suggested that abnormalities in dopamine transmission may be linked to the experience of chronic pain and the accompanying emotional and motivational symptoms.

The neurochemical imbalances in fibromyalgia are not limited to these primary neurotransmitters. Glutamate, an excitatory neurotransmitter, has been found to be elevated in certain brain regions of fibromyalgia patients. High levels of glutamate can lead to increased neuronal excitability and contribute to the central sensitization seen in fibromyalgia. This overactivity of pain pathways can result in the amplification of pain signals and the persistent sensation of pain even in the absence of external stimuli.

Substance P, a neuropeptide involved in pain perception, is also found in higher levels in the cerebrospinal fluid of fibromyalgia patients. Elevated levels of substance P enhance pain transmission and amplify the pain response. This increase is consistent with the enhanced pain sensitivity and widespread pain experienced by fibromyalgia sufferers.

Hormonal Influences

Hormonal influences are a crucial aspect of the complex puzzle that is fibromyalgia, affecting how the body responds to stress, pain, and other stimuli. The endocrine system, which regulates hormones in the body, plays a significant role in maintaining homeostasis and responding to external and internal stressors. In individuals with fibromyalgia, there is growing evidence that hormonal imbalances contribute to the condition's symptoms and severity.

The hypothalamic-pituitary-adrenal (HPA) axis is a central player in the body's stress response system. It involves a series of interactions between the hypothalamus, the pituitary gland, and the adrenal glands. When the body perceives stress, the hypothalamus releases corticotropin-releasing hormone (CRH), which signals the pituitary gland to secrete adrenocorticotropic hormone (ACTH). ACTH then stimulates the adrenal glands to produce cortisol, the primary stress hormone. Cortisol helps the body manage stress by increasing glucose availability, suppressing the immune system, and aiding in metabolism. In fibromyalgia patients, this stress response system is often dysregulated.

Research has shown that individuals with fibromyalgia frequently exhibit abnormal cortisol levels. Some studies have found that fibromyalgia patients have lower-than-normal cortisol levels, which can impair the body's ability to cope with stress. This condition, known as hypocortisolism, can lead to symptoms such as fatigue, weakness, and increased sensitivity to pain. Conversely, other studies have reported elevated nighttime cortisol levels in fibromyalgia patients, which can disrupt sleep patterns and contribute to the non-restorative sleep commonly experienced by those with the condition. This variability in cortisol production highlights the complex nature of the HPA axis dysfunction in fibromyalgia.

In addition to cortisol, other hormones regulated by the HPA axis, such as dehydroepiandrosterone (DHEA), also play a role in fibromyalgia. DHEA serves as a precursor to both estrogen and testosterone and has been shown to have anti-inflammatory and immune-modulating effects. Altered levels of DHEA have been observed in fibromyalgia patients, suggesting that imbalances in this hormone could contribute to the immune dysregulation and inflammation associated with the condition.

Thyroid hormones are another critical aspect of hormonal influence in fibromyalgia. The thyroid gland produces hormones that regulate metabolism, energy levels, and overall metabolic rate. Hypothyroidism, or low thyroid hormone levels, shares many symptoms with fibromyalgia, including fatigue, muscle pain, and cognitive difficulties. Some fibromyalgia patients have been found to have subclinical thyroid dysfunction, where thyroid hormone levels are within the normal range but at the lower end, potentially exacerbating fibromyalgia symptoms. This overlap in symptoms has led researchers to explore the potential link between thyroid function and fibromyalgia, although the exact relationship remains an area of active investigation.

Sex hormones, such as estrogen and progesterone, also play a role in fibromyalgia, particularly in female patients. Many women report that their fibromyalgia symptoms fluctuate with their menstrual cycle, pregnancy, and menopause, suggesting a hormonal component. Estrogen is known to affect pain perception and inflammation, and fluctuations in estrogen levels may influence the severity of fibromyalgia symptoms. Progesterone, which has calming and anti-inflammatory effects, can also impact pain sensitivity and mood. The interaction between these sex hormones and the neurotransmitter systems involved in pain regulation further complicates the hormonal landscape of fibromyalgia.

Insulin and growth hormone, both of which are involved in metabolic processes and tissue repair, have also been implicated in fibromyalgia. Insulin resistance, a condition where cells do not respond effectively to insulin, has been observed in some fibromyalgia patients. This resistance can lead to metabolic disturbances and increased inflammation, contributing to pain and fatigue. Growth hormone, which is essential for tissue growth and repair, is often found at reduced levels in fibromyalgia patients, potentially impairing muscle recovery and contributing to chronic pain.

CHAPTER 2: THE SIGNS & SYMPTOMS

Fibromyalgia manifests through a variety of symptoms, with the most prevalent being widespread musculoskeletal pain. This pain is often described as a persistent, dull ache that affects multiple regions of the body, including the neck, shoulders, back, and hips. Unlike acute pain caused by injury or inflammation, fibromyalgia pain is chronic, typically lasting for months, and does not respond to traditional pain treatments. The pain can vary in intensity, sometimes feeling like a deep, throbbing ache, while at other times it may present as sharp, shooting pains. This variability can be particularly frustrating for those affected, as it makes daily activities unpredictable and challenging.

Fatigue is another hallmark symptom of fibromyalgia, often described as an overwhelming sense of tiredness that is not alleviated by rest or sleep. This fatigue can be so debilitating that it interferes with even the simplest tasks, such as getting out of bed, performing household chores, or maintaining employment. Many individuals with fibromyalgia find that their energy levels are significantly lower than before the onset of their symptoms, leading to a drastic change in lifestyle and activity levels.

Cognitive difficulties, often referred to as "fibro fog," are also common among those with fibromyalgia. These cognitive issues can manifest as problems with concentration, memory, and mental clarity. Individuals may find it challenging to focus on tasks, remember details, or process information efficiently. This can affect both professional and personal aspects of life, making it difficult to perform job-related duties, manage daily schedules, or engage in conversations. The cognitive impairments associated with fibromyalgia can be particularly distressing, as they can lead to a sense of frustration and diminished self-confidence.

Sleep disturbances are another significant component of fibromyalgia. Many patients report difficulty falling asleep, frequent awakenings during the night, and feeling unrefreshed upon waking, a condition known as non-restorative sleep. This lack of quality sleep can exacerbate other symptoms, such as pain and fatigue, creating a vicious cycle that is hard to break. Poor sleep quality can also affect mood and cognitive function, further compounding the challenges faced by individuals with fibromyalgia.

In addition to these primary symptoms, individuals with fibromyalgia often experience heightened sensitivity to various stimuli. This increased sensitivity can include hypersensitivity to pain, known as hyperalgesia, where even mild pressure or touch can cause significant discomfort. Many patients also report heightened sensitivity to temperature changes, light, and sound, making it difficult to tolerate environments that are too hot or cold, brightly lit, or noisy. This hypersensitivity can limit social interactions and participation in activities, contributing to feelings of isolation and frustration.

Less Common Symptoms

In addition to the primary symptoms of fibromyalgia, many individuals experience a range of less common symptoms that can further complicate their condition and overall quality of life. Gastrointestinal issues, such as irritable bowel syndrome (IBS), are frequently reported among fibromyalgia patients. IBS symptoms include abdominal pain, bloating, gas, diarrhea, and constipation, which can vary in intensity and duration. These digestive problems can be particularly distressing, as they add another layer of discomfort and disruption to daily life.

Managing these gastrointestinal symptoms often requires dietary adjustments, medication, and lifestyle changes, further complicating the treatment regimen for fibromyalgia.

Headaches and migraines are also common among individuals with fibromyalgia. These can range from mild tension headaches to severe migraines that include symptoms such as nausea, vomiting, and heightened sensitivity to light and sound. The frequency and intensity of these headaches can significantly impact a person's ability to function, often necessitating additional medications and treatments to manage the pain and associated symptoms. The link between fibromyalgia and migraines underscores the complexity of the condition, as both involve alterations in pain processing pathways.

Temporomandibular joint (TMJ) disorders are another less common symptom experienced by fibromyalgia patients. TMJ disorders cause pain and dysfunction in the jaw joint and the muscles controlling jaw movement. Symptoms can include jaw pain, clicking or popping sounds when opening the mouth, and difficulty chewing or speaking. These issues can interfere with eating, speaking, and other daily activities, contributing to the overall burden of fibromyalgia.

Numbness and tingling sensations, known as paresthesia, can also occur in the hands and feet of those with fibromyalgia. These sensations can range from mild tingling to a more intense, burning feeling. Paresthesia can be particularly bothersome at night, disrupting sleep and leading to further fatigue. Additionally, these sensations can interfere with fine motor skills, making tasks such as typing, buttoning clothes, or handling small objects more difficult.

Restless legs syndrome (RLS) is another condition that commonly co-occurs with fibromyalgia. RLS is characterized by an uncontrollable urge to move the legs, often accompanied by uncomfortable sensations such as itching, tingling, or creeping feelings. These symptoms typically worsen in the evening or at night, making it difficult to fall asleep and stay asleep. The resulting sleep disturbances can exacerbate the fatigue and cognitive difficulties associated with fibromyalgia, creating a challenging cycle of symptoms.

Other less common symptoms of fibromyalgia include hypersensitivity to environmental factors, such as bright lights, loud noises, and strong smells. This heightened sensitivity can make everyday environments overwhelming and uncomfortable, limiting social interactions and participation in activities. Additionally, some individuals with fibromyalgia may experience dizziness, balance issues, and coordination problems, which can increase the risk of falls and injuries.

Depression and anxiety are also prevalent among fibromyalgia patients, often stemming from the chronic nature of the condition and the constant struggle to manage symptoms. These mood disorders can further complicate the clinical picture of fibromyalgia, as they can amplify the perception of pain and fatigue, and hinder effective coping strategies. Treating depression and anxiety in fibromyalgia patients often requires a multifaceted approach, including medication, therapy, and lifestyle interventions.

Symptom Variability

One of the most challenging aspects of living with fibromyalgia is the unpredictable variability of symptoms. Unlike many other chronic conditions where symptoms remain relatively stable or follow a predictable pattern, fibromyalgia symptoms can fluctuate dramatically from day to day or even hour to hour. This unpredictability makes it difficult for individuals to plan and carry out daily activities, as they cannot anticipate how they will feel at any given time. Factors such as physical activity, stress, weather changes, and sleep quality can all influence the severity and occurrence of symptoms, creating a complex and often overwhelming experience for those affected.

The variability of symptoms means that individuals with fibromyalgia must constantly adapt their routines and expectations. On some days, they may feel relatively well and capable of engaging in work, social activities, and exercise. On other days, they may be so overwhelmed by pain, fatigue, and cognitive difficulties that even simple tasks like getting out of bed or taking a shower become insurmountable challenges. This inconsistency can lead to a significant reduction in productivity and participation in daily life, contributing to feelings of frustration, helplessness, and social isolation.

The impact of symptom variability extends to every aspect of life. For those who are employed, managing a job can become a monumental task. The cognitive impairments, often referred to as "fibro fog," can affect memory, concentration, and the ability to process information, making it difficult to perform job-related duties efficiently. Frequent absences due to severe flare-ups can jeopardize job security and career advancement. This uncertainty can also strain relationships with colleagues and supervisors, who may not fully understand the nature of the condition and its impact on performance.

In personal and social spheres, the unpredictable nature of fibromyalgia symptoms can disrupt relationships with family and friends. Plans may need to be canceled or rescheduled at the last minute due to sudden flare-ups, leading to feelings of guilt and frustration. Loved ones may struggle to comprehend the invisible and fluctuating nature of the illness, sometimes leading to misunderstandings and a lack of support. The social isolation that can result from these dynamics further exacerbates the emotional burden of living with fibromyalgia.

Symptom variability also affects physical health and fitness. Regular exercise is often recommended as a way to manage fibromyalgia symptoms, but the pain and fatigue associated with the condition can make it challenging to maintain a consistent exercise routine. On good days, individuals may be able to engage in physical activity, but overexertion can lead to increased pain and fatigue on subsequent days, creating a cycle of boom and bust that hinders progress and discourages regular exercise. This inconsistency can result in a decline in overall physical health and contribute to the deconditioning often seen in fibromyalgia patients.

The emotional toll of symptom variability is profound. The constant uncertainty about how one will feel can lead to chronic stress and anxiety. The fear of experiencing a severe flare-up can cause individuals to avoid activities and situations that they might otherwise enjoy, further limiting their quality of life. Depression is also common among those with fibromyalgia, often stemming from the relentless and unpredictable nature of the condition.

CHAPTER 3: GETTING DIAGNOSED

Diagnosing fibromyalgia can be a complex and nuanced process, as the condition lacks a definitive test and is characterized by a wide range of symptoms that overlap with other disorders. The diagnostic criteria for fibromyalgia have evolved over the years as our understanding of the disorder has deepened. Historically, the American College of Rheumatology (ACR) set the initial criteria in 1990, which focused primarily on the presence of widespread pain and tenderness at specific points on the body. However, these criteria have been updated to reflect a more comprehensive understanding of fibromyalgia, encompassing a broader range of symptoms.

The 1990 ACR criteria required that a patient experience widespread pain for at least three months, with pain present in all four quadrants of the body: both sides and above and below the waist. Additionally, the patient needed to exhibit tenderness in at least 11 of 18 specific tender points when pressure was applied. These tender points included areas such as the back of the head, tops of the shoulders, outer elbows, upper hips, sides of the hips, and knees. While these criteria were a significant step forward, they were somewhat limited as they focused heavily on the tender point examination and did not account for the range of other symptoms experienced by those with fibromyalgia.

In 2010, the ACR updated the diagnostic criteria to better capture the full spectrum of fibromyalgia symptoms. The new criteria moved away from the tender point count and introduced the Widespread Pain Index (WPI) and the Symptom Severity Scale (SSS). The WPI assesses the number of body regions where the patient has experienced pain over the past week. Specifically, it involves identifying up to 19 areas where pain is felt, including regions such as the shoulders, arms, legs, chest, abdomen, and back. Each area where pain is present contributes to the overall WPI score, which can range from 0 to 19.

The Symptom Severity Scale (SSS) evaluates the severity of three key symptoms: fatigue, waking unrefreshed, and cognitive difficulties (often referred to as "fibro fog"). Each of these symptoms is scored on a scale from 0 to 3, with 0 indicating no problem and 3 indicating severe, pervasive problems. Additionally, the SSS includes an assessment of the presence and severity of other somatic symptoms, such as headaches, depression, anxiety, and irritable bowel syndrome. These symptoms are scored on a scale from 0 to 12, contributing to an overall SSS score that can range from 0 to 12.

To meet the updated 2010 ACR criteria for fibromyalgia, a patient must have a WPI score of 7 or higher and an SSS score of 5 or higher, or a WPI score between 3 and 6 and an SSS score of 9 or higher. This approach allows for a more nuanced assessment of the patient's symptomatology, capturing the widespread pain and the multi-faceted nature of the condition.

In 2016, the ACR further refined the criteria to simplify the diagnostic process and improve its accuracy. These revised criteria include the same WPI and SSS components but emphasize the necessity of symptom persistence. Specifically, the criteria require that the symptoms have been present at a similar level for at least three months, ensuring that transient or acute pain conditions are not misdiagnosed as fibromyalgia. Additionally, the criteria require that there is no other disorder that would otherwise explain the pain and symptoms experienced by the patient.

Similar Conditions

Diagnosing fibromyalgia involves not only identifying its specific symptoms but also ruling out other conditions that can present with similar features. This process is crucial because many disorders share overlapping symptoms with fibromyalgia, making differential diagnosis a key component of the evaluation. Understanding these similar or co-morbid conditions helps ensure an accurate diagnosis and appropriate treatment plan

One of the primary conditions that must be ruled out is rheumatoid arthritis (RA). RA is an autoimmune disorder that primarily affects the joints, causing inflammation, pain, and swelling. Like fibromyalgia, RA can lead to significant pain and fatigue. However, RA typically presents with more pronounced joint swelling and deformities, which are less common in fibromyalgia. Blood tests for rheumatoid factor (RF) and anti-citrullinated protein antibodies (ACPAs) are used to detect RA. Elevated levels of these antibodies, along with imaging studies showing joint erosion, can help distinguish RA from fibromyalgia.

Lupus, another autoimmune disease, also shares symptoms with fibromyalgia, such as widespread pain, fatigue, and cognitive difficulties. However, lupus often involves additional symptoms like a characteristic butterfly-shaped rash across the cheeks and nose, photosensitivity, and organ involvement (e.g., kidneys, heart). Antinuclear antibody (ANA) testing, along with other specific autoantibodies (e.g., anti-dsDNA, anti-Smith), can help diagnose lupus. A comprehensive evaluation of symptoms, clinical history, and laboratory results is necessary to differentiate lupus from fibromyalgia.

Multiple sclerosis (MS) is a neurological condition that can mimic some fibromyalgia symptoms, particularly fatigue, cognitive dysfunction, and pain. MS involves the immune system attacking the protective covering of nerves, leading to communication problems between the brain and the rest of the body. Symptoms like muscle weakness, vision problems, and balance issues are more specific to MS. Magnetic resonance imaging (MRI) of the brain and spinal cord, along with cerebrospinal fluid analysis, are critical in diagnosing MS and differentiating it from fibromyalgia.

Chronic fatigue syndrome (CFS), also known as myalgic encephalomyelitis (ME), is another condition with significant symptom overlap with fibromyalgia, including profound fatigue, sleep disturbances, and cognitive impairments. One distinguishing feature of CFS is post-exertional malaise (PEM), where symptoms worsen after physical or mental exertion and can last for days or weeks. There is no specific test for CFS, but diagnosis involves a thorough evaluation of symptoms and exclusion of other medical conditions. The differentiation between fibromyalgia and CFS can be subtle, and some patients may have both conditions.

Hypothyroidism, or underactive thyroid, is characterized by fatigue, muscle pain, and cognitive issues, which can easily be mistaken for fibromyalgia. However, hypothyroidism typically presents with additional symptoms such as weight gain, cold intolerance, dry skin, and hair loss. Blood tests measuring thyroid-stimulating hormone (TSH) and free thyroxine (T4) levels are essential for diagnosing hypothyroidism. Normal thyroid function tests can help exclude hypothyroidism as the cause of the symptoms.

Irritable bowel syndrome (IBS) often coexists with fibromyalgia and shares symptoms such as abdominal pain, bloating, and altered bowel habits. While IBS is a gastrointestinal disorder, its presence can complicate the clinical picture of fibromyalgia. Diagnosis of IBS is based on clinical criteria, such as the Rome IV criteria, which include recurrent abdominal pain associated with defecation or changes in stool frequency and form. Managing IBS symptoms can be an integral part of fibromyalgia treatment.

Temporomandibular joint (TMJ) disorders cause pain and dysfunction in the jaw joint and muscles, which can overlap with fibromyalgia symptoms. TMJ disorders can present with jaw pain, headaches, and earaches. A thorough dental examination, imaging studies, and evaluation by a specialist in TMJ disorders can help distinguish these issues from fibromyalgia-related pain.

Depression and anxiety are common comorbid conditions with fibromyalgia, and their symptoms can overlap significantly, including fatigue, sleep disturbances, and cognitive difficulties. A comprehensive psychological evaluation can help identify these mental health conditions, which may require concurrent treatment alongside fibromyalgia management.

Sleep disorders, such as obstructive sleep apnea (OSA) and restless legs syndrome (RLS), also need to be ruled out. OSA involves repeated episodes of blocked breathing during sleep, leading to poor sleep quality and daytime fatigue. RLS causes an uncontrollable urge to move the legs, often accompanied by uncomfortable sensations, particularly at night. Sleep studies (polysomnography) can diagnose these conditions, which, if treated, may alleviate some of the symptoms attributed to fibromyalgia.

Other conditions that may mimic fibromyalgia symptoms include polymyalgia rheumatica, Lyme disease, and certain infections (e.g., hepatitis, HIV). Polymyalgia rheumatica presents with muscle pain and stiffness, particularly in the shoulders and hips, and is often associated with elevated inflammatory markers. Lyme disease, caused by the Borrelia burgdorferi bacterium, can lead to widespread pain and fatigue, and is diagnosed through a combination of clinical presentation and laboratory tests. Infections like hepatitis and HIV can cause systemic symptoms that overlap with fibromyalgia, necessitating appropriate screening tests.

Challenges in Diagnosing Fibromyalgia

Diagnosing fibromyalgia presents numerous challenges for both patients and healthcare providers, primarily due to the condition's complex and multifaceted nature. One of the most significant challenges is the lack of a definitive diagnostic test. Unlike conditions such as diabetes or rheumatoid arthritis, which can be confirmed through blood tests or imaging studies, fibromyalgia does not have a specific biomarker or test that can conclusively diagnose it. Instead, diagnosis relies heavily on clinical criteria and the exclusion of other potential conditions, making the process inherently subjective and often protracted.

The variability of symptoms in fibromyalgia adds another layer of complexity to the diagnostic process. Patients may experience a wide range of symptoms, including chronic widespread pain, fatigue, cognitive difficulties, and sleep disturbances, but these symptoms can fluctuate in intensity and frequency. This variability can make it difficult for healthcare providers to identify a consistent pattern that fits the diagnostic criteria for fibromyalgia. Additionally, symptoms may overlap with those of other conditions, further complicating the differential diagnosis.

The subjective nature of fibromyalgia symptoms also poses a significant challenge. Pain, fatigue, and cognitive difficulties are inherently subjective experiences that rely on patient self-reporting. This subjectivity can make it challenging for healthcare providers to objectively measure and evaluate the severity of symptoms. Patients may have difficulty articulating their experiences, and the fluctuating nature of symptoms can lead to inconsistent descriptions from one medical visit to another.

Another major challenge in diagnosing fibromyalgia is the widespread stigma and misunderstanding surrounding the condition. Despite advances in medical understanding, fibromyalgia is still sometimes viewed with skepticism by both healthcare providers and the general public. Some providers may dismiss fibromyalgia symptoms as psychosomatic or attribute them to anxiety or depression, rather than recognizing fibromyalgia as a legitimate medical condition. This skepticism can lead to delays in diagnosis, inadequate treatment, and significant frustration for patients who are seeking validation and relief for their symptoms.

Patients often face a long and arduous journey to diagnosis, seeing multiple healthcare providers over several years. This process can involve extensive testing to rule out other conditions, repeated misdiagnoses, and ineffective treatments. The emotional and psychological toll of this prolonged diagnostic journey can be substantial, contributing to feelings of hopelessness and distress. For many patients, the lack of a clear diagnosis can impact their quality of life, affecting their ability to work, maintain relationships, and engage in daily activities. Research indicates that fibromyalgia often goes undiagnosed or misdiagnosed. Studies suggest that a significant percentage of fibromyalgia cases are missed, with estimates indicating that up to 75% of people with fibromyalgia may remain undiagnosed. Additionally, it is not uncommon for fibromyalgia to be misdiagnosed as other conditions, such as chronic fatigue syndrome, depression, or rheumatoid arthritis, further complicating the treatment process.

Healthcare providers also face challenges in diagnosing fibromyalgia due to the need for comprehensive and detailed patient evaluations. Conducting a thorough assessment requires significant time and attention, which can be difficult to manage in a busy clinical setting. Providers must take a holistic approach, considering the patient's medical history, symptom presentation, and the impact of symptoms on daily life. They must also be knowledgeable about the latest diagnostic criteria and guidelines to ensure an accurate and timely diagnosis.

Effective communication between patients and healthcare providers is crucial in overcoming these challenges. Patients need to feel comfortable discussing their symptoms in detail, and providers must listen actively and empathetically to understand the full scope of the patient's experience. Building a trusting relationship is essential for accurately assessing symptoms and developing an effective treatment plan.

Who to See to Receive a Diagnosis

If you suspect you have fibromyalgia, the first step is to consult with a primary care physician. Primary care doctors, such as family physicians or internists, can perform an initial evaluation, review your medical history, and conduct a physical examination. They are well-equipped to order preliminary tests to rule out other conditions that might be causing your symptoms. If fibromyalgia is suspected, your primary care physician can guide you through the next steps and refer you to a specialist for further evaluation.

Rheumatologists are often the specialists most knowledgeable about fibromyalgia and are frequently involved in diagnosing and managing the condition. Rheumatologists specialize in musculoskeletal diseases and autoimmune disorders, making them well-suited to differentiate fibromyalgia from other similar conditions such as rheumatoid arthritis and lupus. A rheumatologist can provide a comprehensive evaluation, including a detailed medical history, physical examination, and any necessary laboratory tests or imaging studies to confirm the diagnosis and rule out other disorders.

Neurologists are another type of specialist who may be consulted, particularly if you have significant neurological symptoms such as severe cognitive difficulties, headaches, or numbness and tingling sensations. Neurologists specialize in disorders of the nervous system and can conduct a thorough neurological examination. They may order tests such as MRI scans or nerve conduction studies to ensure that there are no underlying neurological conditions contributing to your symptoms.

Pain management specialists, also known as pain physicians, focus on the diagnosis and treatment of chronic pain conditions. These specialists can provide a comprehensive approach to managing fibromyalgia pain through a variety of treatments, including medications, physical therapy, and interventional procedures. Pain management specialists can work in conjunction with other healthcare providers to create a multidisciplinary treatment plan tailored to your specific needs.

Sleep specialists may be consulted if sleep disturbances are a prominent feature of your fibromyalgia symptoms. Sleep specialists are trained to diagnose and treat sleep disorders, such as sleep apnea and restless legs syndrome, which are commonly associated with fibromyalgia. A sleep study, or polysomnography, may be conducted to assess your sleep patterns and identify any sleep-related issues that need to be addressed as part of your overall treatment plan.

Psychiatrists and psychologists can also play an important role in the diagnosis and management of fibromyalgia, particularly if you are experiencing significant mental health symptoms such as depression, anxiety, or stress. These mental health professionals can provide counseling, cognitive-behavioral therapy (CBT), and other therapeutic interventions to help you cope with the emotional and psychological impact of fibromyalgia. They can also collaborate with other healthcare providers to ensure that your treatment plan addresses both physical and mental health needs.

When seeking a diagnosis for fibromyalgia, it is crucial to find healthcare providers who are knowledgeable, compassionate, and experienced in managing the condition. Given the complexity and subjective nature of fibromyalgia symptoms, a supportive and understanding medical team can make a significant difference in the diagnostic process and ongoing management. It may be helpful to seek recommendations from support groups, patient advocacy organizations, or online communities to find providers with expertise in fibromyalgia.

CHAPTER 4: TREATING FIBROMYALGIA WITH MEDICATION

Treating fibromyalgia often requires a comprehensive approach, and medications can play a crucial role in managing the symptoms. Various medications are commonly prescribed to help alleviate the pain, fatigue, and cognitive difficulties associated with fibromyalgia. In this chapter, we will explore the different types of medications that are commonly prescribed, their brand names, how they work, and their potential side effects.

Antidepressants

Amitriptyline (Brand Name: Elavil)

Amitriptyline is a tricyclic antidepressant that helps increase the levels of neurotransmitters in the brain, such as serotonin and norepinephrine, which can help reduce pain and improve sleep. It is often prescribed in low doses for fibromyalgia.

Potential Side Effects: Drowsiness, dry mouth, constipation, weight gain, blurred vision, and urinary retention.

Duloxetine (Brand Name: Cymbalta)

Duloxetine is a serotonin-norepinephrine reuptake inhibitor (SNRI) that can help reduce pain and improve mood by increasing the levels of serotonin and norepinephrine in the brain.

Potential Side Effects: Nausea, dry mouth, constipation, loss of appetite, fatigue, and increased sweating.

Milnacipran (Brand Name: Savella)

Milnacipran is another SNRI specifically approved for the treatment of fibromyalgia. It works by increasing the levels of serotonin and norepinephrine, which can help alleviate pain and improve overall function.

Potential Side Effects: Nausea, headache, constipation, dizziness, insomnia, and increased heart rate.

Fluoxetine (Brand Name: Prozac)

Fluoxetine is a selective serotonin reuptake inhibitor (SSRI) that can help improve mood and reduce pain. It is sometimes used in combination with other medications for fibromyalgia.

Potential Side Effects: Nausea, insomnia, drowsiness, anxiety, and sexual dysfunction.

Anticonvulsants

Pregabalin (Brand Name: Lyrica)

Pregabalin is an anticonvulsant that helps reduce pain by decreasing the release of certain neurotransmitters involved in pain signaling. It is specifically approved for the treatment of fibromyalgia.

Potential Side Effects: Dizziness, drowsiness, weight gain, blurred vision, dry mouth, and swelling in the hands and feet.

Gabapentin (Brand Name: Neurontin)

Gabapentin is another anticonvulsant that is commonly used off-label for fibromyalgia. It works similarly to pregabalin by reducing the release of neurotransmitters that contribute to pain.

Potential Side Effects: Dizziness, drowsiness, peripheral edema, weight gain, and difficulty concentrating.

Pain Relievers

Tramadol (Brand Name: Ultram)

Tramadol is an opioid-like pain reliever that can help manage moderate to severe pain in fibromyalgia patients. It works by binding to opioid receptors and inhibiting the reuptake of serotonin and norepinephrine.

Potential Side Effects: Nausea, dizziness, constipation, headache, drowsiness, and risk of dependence and withdrawal symptoms.

Acetaminophen (Brand Name: Tylenol)

Acetaminophen is an over-the-counter pain reliever that can help manage mild to moderate pain in fibromyalgia patients. It is often used in combination with other medications for more comprehensive pain management.

Potential Side Effects: Generally well-tolerated, but high doses can cause liver damage.

Muscle Relaxants

Cyclobenzaprine (Brand Name: Flexeril)

Cyclobenzaprine is a muscle relaxant that can help reduce muscle spasms and improve sleep quality in fibromyalgia patients. It is often used in conjunction with other medications.

Potential Side Effects: Drowsiness, dry mouth, dizziness, and constipation.

Sleep Aids

Zolpidem (Brand Name: Ambien)

Zolpidem is a sedative-hypnotic medication that can help improve sleep quality in patients with fibromyalgia who have difficulty falling asleep or staying asleep.

Potential Side Effects: Drowsiness, dizziness, headache, and potential for dependence and unusual sleep behaviors.

Anti-Inflammatories

Nonsteroidal Anti-Inflammatory Drugs (NSAIDs)

NSAIDs, such as ibuprofen (Brand Name: Advil, Motrin) and naproxen (Brand Name: Aleve), can help manage pain and inflammation in some fibromyalgia patients. However, they are generally less effective for fibromyalgia pain compared to other conditions involving inflammation.

Potential Side Effects: Stomach upset, gastrointestinal bleeding, kidney issues, and increased risk of heart problems with long-term use.

Anti-Anxiety Medications

Benzodiazepines (e.g., Clonazepam - Brand Name: Klonopin)

Benzodiazepines can help manage anxiety and improve sleep quality in fibromyalgia patients. They are usually prescribed for short-term use due to the risk of dependence.

Potential Side Effects: Drowsiness, dizziness, confusion, and potential for dependence and withdrawal symptoms.

Other Medications

Low-Dose Naltrexone (LDN)

Low-dose naltrexone is an off-label treatment that some studies suggest may help reduce pain and improve quality of life in fibromyalgia patients. It works by modulating the immune system and reducing inflammation.

Potential Side Effects: Vivid dreams, insomnia, headache, and gastrointestinal discomfort.

CHAPTER 5: ADDITIONAL TREATMENT OPTIONS

While medications can play a critical role in managing fibromyalgia symptoms, a comprehensive treatment plan often includes various other therapies to address the wide range of symptoms experienced by patients. This chapter explores the different non-pharmacological treatments that may be prescribed to help alleviate pain, improve function, and enhance the overall quality of life for individuals with fibromyalgia.

Physical Therapy

Physical therapy (PT) is a cornerstone of fibromyalgia management and can significantly improve the quality of life for those living with the condition. Physical therapists are healthcare professionals who specialize in evaluating and treating physical impairments, disabilities, and conditions through targeted exercise and manual therapy techniques. When it comes to fibromyalgia, the primary goals of physical therapy are to reduce pain, improve mobility, enhance strength, and increase overall function.

One of the main components of a physical therapy program for fibromyalgia is the development of a personalized exercise regimen. This regimen typically includes low-impact aerobic exercises such as swimming, walking, and cycling. These activities are chosen because they are gentle on the joints and muscles, reducing the risk of exacerbating pain while improving cardiovascular health. Aerobic exercise helps increase stamina, reduce fatigue, and boost mood by promoting the release of endorphins, the body's natural painkillers.

Strength training exercises are another critical element of physical therapy for fibromyalgia. These exercises focus on building muscle strength and endurance, which can help support the joints and reduce the overall burden on the body. Strength training exercises are often performed using resistance bands, free weights, or bodyweight exercises. Physical therapists ensure that these exercises are tailored to the individual's fitness level, starting with low resistance and gradually increasing as tolerated to avoid overexertion and flare-ups.

Flexibility and stretching exercises are also integral to a physical therapy program for fibromyalgia. These exercises help to reduce muscle stiffness, improve range of motion, and prevent the formation of painful muscle knots or trigger points. Stretching routines may include static stretches, where a stretch is held for a specific duration, and dynamic stretches, which involve moving parts of the body through a range of motion. Physical therapists guide patients through these exercises, emphasizing proper technique and breathing to maximize the benefits.

Manual therapy techniques, such as massage and myofascial release, are often incorporated into physical therapy sessions to address muscle tension and pain. These hands-on techniques involve the physical therapist applying controlled pressure to specific areas of the body to release tight muscles and fascia (the connective tissue surrounding muscles). Manual therapy can help improve circulation, reduce muscle spasms, and enhance overall mobility.

Another important aspect of physical therapy for fibromyalgia is patient education. Physical therapists educate patients about body mechanics and ergonomics, which are essential for minimizing strain and preventing injury during daily activities. This education includes teaching proper posture, lifting techniques, and ways to modify activities to reduce the risk of pain and flare-ups. Patients learn how to recognize and respond to their body's signals, pacing themselves to avoid overexertion and allowing adequate rest and recovery.

Physical therapists also use modalities such as heat and cold therapy, ultrasound, and transcutaneous electrical nerve stimulation (TENS) to manage pain and inflammation. Heat therapy involves applying warm packs or using heat wraps to relax muscles and improve blood flow, while cold therapy uses ice packs to reduce inflammation and numb painful areas. Ultrasound therapy uses sound waves to generate heat deep within tissues, promoting healing and reducing pain. TENS involves the use of low-voltage electrical currents to stimulate nerves and disrupt pain signals, providing temporary pain relief.

Balance and coordination exercises may also be included in a physical therapy program for fibromyalgia. These exercises help improve proprioception (the body's ability to sense its position in space) and reduce the risk of falls and injuries. Balance training might involve exercises like standing on one leg, using a balance board, or performing specific movements that challenge stability.

Throughout the physical therapy process, physical therapists continuously assess and adjust the treatment plan based on the patient's progress and feedback. This individualized approach ensures that the therapy remains effective and responsive to the patient's changing needs. Physical therapists work closely with other healthcare providers, such as rheumatologists, pain specialists, and primary care physicians, to provide a coordinated and comprehensive treatment plan.

Myotherapy

Myotherapy, also known as trigger point therapy, is a specialized form of manual therapy aimed at relieving pain and dysfunction in the musculoskeletal system by targeting specific trigger points. These trigger points are hyperirritable spots within taut bands of muscle fibers that can cause localized pain and referred pain in other parts of the body. Myotherapy is particularly beneficial for individuals with fibromyalgia, as it addresses muscle pain and tension, which are common symptoms of the condition.

Myotherapists are trained professionals who utilize a variety of techniques to deactivate trigger points and alleviate muscle tightness. The therapy typically begins with a comprehensive assessment to identify the location and severity of trigger points. This assessment involves palpation of the muscles and detailed questioning about the patient's pain patterns, daily activities, and medical history. Understanding the patient's unique pain profile allows the myotherapist to tailor the treatment plan to their specific needs.

One of the primary techniques used in myotherapy is direct pressure. The myotherapist applies sustained pressure to the trigger point using their fingers, knuckles, or specialized tools. This pressure may be initially uncomfortable but is usually followed by a sense of relief as the muscle fibers begin to relax. The duration and intensity of the pressure are carefully controlled to ensure effectiveness while minimizing discomfort. The goal is to disrupt the pain cycle, increase blood flow to the area, and promote the release of tension.

In addition to direct pressure, myotherapy may include other manual techniques such as stretching, massage, and myofascial release. Stretching helps elongate the muscle fibers, reducing tension and improving flexibility. Specific stretches targeting affected muscle groups can be incorporated into the therapy sessions, with the myotherapist guiding the patient through each movement to ensure proper technique and prevent injury.

Massage techniques used in myotherapy range from gentle strokes to deep tissue manipulation. These techniques help to relax the muscles, enhance circulation, and reduce pain and stiffness. Myofascial release focuses on the fascia, the connective tissue that surrounds and supports the muscles. By applying gentle, sustained pressure, myofascial release aims to relieve restrictions in the fascia, which can contribute to pain and dysfunction.

Another component of myotherapy is corrective exercise. Myotherapists may prescribe specific exercises to strengthen weak muscles, improve posture, and enhance overall musculoskeletal health. These exercises are designed to complement the manual therapy techniques and provide long-term benefits by addressing underlying imbalances and preventing the recurrence of trigger points. Patients are taught how to perform these exercises correctly and are encouraged to incorporate them into their daily routines.

Heat therapy is often used in conjunction with myotherapy to further relax muscles and increase blood flow. Warm packs or heat wraps may be applied to the affected areas before or after the manual techniques to enhance their effectiveness. Heat therapy can help reduce muscle stiffness, making it easier to release trigger points and alleviate pain.

Education and self-care are integral parts of myotherapy. Myotherapists provide patients with information on how to manage their symptoms between sessions. This may include advice on proper ergonomics, posture, and body mechanics to minimize strain on the muscles. Patients are also taught self-massage techniques and stretching exercises that they can perform at home to maintain the benefits of the therapy and prevent the recurrence of trigger points.

The benefits of myotherapy for fibromyalgia patients are multifaceted. By targeting trigger points and relieving muscle tension, myotherapy can significantly reduce pain and improve mobility. Patients often report a decrease in muscle stiffness and an increase in flexibility and range of motion. The relaxation induced by myotherapy can also have a positive impact on sleep quality and overall well-being, which are often compromised in individuals with fibromyalgia.

Chiropractic Care

Chiropractic care is a holistic approach to health that focuses on diagnosing and treating musculoskeletal disorders, particularly those involving the spine. Chiropractors use manual manipulation and adjustment techniques to improve spinal alignment and overall musculoskeletal function. For individuals with fibromyalgia, chiropractic care can be an effective component of a comprehensive treatment plan, addressing pain, improving mobility, and enhancing overall well-being.

Chiropractic care begins with a thorough assessment of the patient's medical history, symptoms, and physical condition. This assessment often includes a detailed examination of the spine, posture, and range of motion, as well as discussions about the patient's lifestyle, daily activities, and specific health concerns. Chiropractors may also use diagnostic imaging, such as X-rays or MRIs, to gain a better understanding of the patient's spinal health and identify any structural issues that may be contributing to their symptoms.

The core technique used in chiropractic care is spinal manipulation, also known as spinal adjustment. During a spinal adjustment, the chiropractor uses their hands or a specialized instrument to apply controlled, sudden force to a specific joint in the spine. This technique aims to restore proper alignment, improve joint mobility, and alleviate pain. For fibromyalgia patients, spinal adjustments can help reduce muscle tension, decrease nerve irritation, and enhance the body's natural ability to heal.

In addition to spinal manipulation, chiropractors often use other manual therapy techniques to address fibromyalgia symptoms. These techniques may include soft tissue therapy, such as massage or myofascial release, to relax tight muscles, improve circulation, and reduce pain. Soft tissue therapy can be particularly beneficial for fibromyalgia patients who experience widespread muscle tenderness and stiffness. Chiropractors may also incorporate stretching and mobilization techniques to improve flexibility and range of motion in affected areas.

Chiropractic care often includes recommendations for lifestyle modifications and self-care practices that support overall health and well-being. Chiropractors provide guidance on ergonomics, posture, and body mechanics to help patients minimize strain and prevent injury during daily activities. They may suggest specific exercises to strengthen muscles, improve balance, and enhance physical function. These exercises are tailored to the individual's needs and abilities, ensuring they are safe and effective for managing fibromyalgia symptoms.

One of the benefits of chiropractic care for fibromyalgia patients is its holistic approach, which considers the interconnectedness of the body's systems. Chiropractors recognize that fibromyalgia affects not only the musculoskeletal system but also the nervous system and overall health. By addressing the underlying structural issues and promoting optimal spinal health, chiropractic care can help reduce pain, improve physical function, and enhance the body's resilience to stress.

Chiropractic care can also include the use of adjunct therapies to support the primary treatment. These therapies may include heat and cold therapy, ultrasound, and electrical stimulation. Heat therapy involves applying warm packs to the affected areas to relax muscles and increase blood flow, while cold therapy uses ice packs to reduce inflammation and numb pain. Ultrasound therapy uses sound waves to penetrate deep into tissues, promoting healing and reducing pain. Electrical stimulation, such as transcutaneous electrical nerve stimulation (TENS), involves using low-voltage electrical currents to stimulate nerves and disrupt pain signals.

Chiropractors often take a multidisciplinary approach to fibromyalgia management, collaborating with other healthcare providers such as primary care physicians, rheumatologists, physical therapists, and nutritionists. This collaborative approach ensures that patients receive comprehensive care that addresses all aspects of their condition.

Injections

Injections are sometimes used as part of a comprehensive treatment plan for fibromyalgia to help manage pain and inflammation. These treatments can provide targeted relief to specific areas of the body, offering benefits that oral medications may not. While injections are not a primary treatment for fibromyalgia, they can be an effective adjunct therapy for some patients. Corticosteroid injections, also known as steroid injections, are commonly used to reduce inflammation and alleviate pain in specific areas. These injections contain corticosteroids, which are powerful anti-inflammatory medications. When injected directly into a painful or inflamed area, such as a joint or muscle, corticosteroids can help decrease swelling and reduce pain. For fibromyalgia patients, corticosteroid injections may be used to target particularly troublesome areas where inflammation and pain are concentrated, such as the shoulders, hips, or knees. The procedure for administering corticosteroid injections involves cleaning the injection site, using a local anesthetic to numb the area, and then injecting the corticosteroid medication. The effects of the injection can last from several weeks to several months, providing temporary relief and allowing patients to engage more comfortably in physical therapy and other treatments. However, corticosteroid injections are typically limited to a few times a year to avoid potential side effects such as tissue damage, weakening of tendons, and increased risk of infection.

Trigger point injections are another type of injection therapy used to manage fibromyalgia symptoms. Trigger points are hyperirritable spots within taut bands of muscle that can cause localized and referred pain. These points can be particularly problematic for fibromyalgia patients, contributing to widespread muscle pain and tenderness. Trigger point injections involve injecting a small amount of local anesthetic, saline, or corticosteroid directly into the trigger point to alleviate pain and relax the muscle. The procedure for trigger point injections is relatively straightforward. The healthcare provider identifies the trigger point through palpation, cleans the area, and then uses a fine needle to inject the medication into the muscle knot. The injection can provide immediate pain relief by disrupting the pain signal and reducing muscle spasms. Patients may experience some discomfort during the procedure, but it is usually brief. Trigger point injections can be repeated as needed, depending on the severity and recurrence of the trigger point s.

Botulinum toxin injections, commonly known by the brand name Botox, are another option for managing certain types of pain associated with fibromyalgia. Botox is a neurotoxin that temporarily paralyzes muscles by blocking the release of acetylcholine, a neurotransmitter that triggers muscle contractions. By injecting Botox into specific muscles, healthcare providers can reduce muscle spasms and pain. Botox injections are typically used for treating chronic migraines and other muscle-related pain conditions. For fibromyalgia patients, Botox may be considered if they experience severe muscle spasms or chronic headaches that do not respond to other treatments. The procedure involves injecting small amounts of Botox into the affected muscles, with effects lasting for several months. Patients may need repeated injections to maintain symptom relief. Potential side effects include localized pain, swelling, and muscle weakness at the injection site.

Prolotherapy, short for proliferative therapy, is an injection-based treatment aimed at promoting the healing of injured or weakened tissues. It involves injecting a solution, often containing dextrose or another irritant, into the affected ligaments, tendons, or joints. The injection stimulates the body's natural healing response, promoting the growth of new tissue and strengthening the area. For fibromyalgia patients, prolotherapy may be used to address joint pain and instability that contributes to their overall discomfort. The procedure involves multiple injections over a series of treatment sessions. While prolotherapy is considered safe, its efficacy for fibromyalgia is still under investigation, and more research is needed to determine its long-term benefits.

Hyaluronic acid injections, also known as viscosupplementation, are used to treat joint pain, particularly in the knees. Hyaluronic acid is a naturally occurring substance in joint fluid that helps lubricate and cushion the joint. In patients with fibromyalgia who also suffer from osteoarthritis or joint degeneration, hyaluronic acid injections can help reduce pain and improve joint function. The procedure involves injecting hyaluronic acid directly into the joint space, usually in a series of injections over several weeks. The effects can last for several months, providing long-term relief and improving the patient's ability to participate in physical activities. Potential side effects include temporary pain, swelling, and stiffness at the injection site.

While injections can provide significant relief for fibromyalgia patients, they are not without risks. Potential side effects vary depending on the type of injection but may include infection, bleeding, allergic reactions, and localized pain or swelling. It is essential for patients to discuss the potential benefits and risks of injection therapy with their healthcare provider to make an informed decision.

Massage Therapy

Massage therapy is a widely used treatment for managing the symptoms of fibromyalgia, offering numerous benefits such as pain relief, muscle relaxation, and stress reduction. As a hands-on therapy, massage involves the manipulation of soft tissues, including muscles, tendons, and ligaments, to alleviate tension and improve circulation. For individuals with fibromyalgia, regular massage therapy sessions can play a crucial role in enhancing overall well-being and quality of life.

The primary goal of massage therapy for fibromyalgia patients is to reduce muscle pain and stiffness. Fibromyalgia often causes widespread musculoskeletal pain, which can lead to tight and tender muscles. Massage therapy helps to release this tension by applying various techniques tailored to the patient's needs. One common technique is Swedish massage, which uses long, gliding strokes, kneading, and circular movements to promote relaxation and improve blood flow. This gentle approach is particularly beneficial for fibromyalgia patients, as it can help alleviate pain without causing additional discomfort.

Deep tissue massage is another technique that may be used for fibromyalgia patients, although it requires careful consideration due to the intensity of the pressure applied. Deep tissue massage targets deeper layers of muscle and connective tissue, aiming to break down adhesions and alleviate chronic muscle tension. While this type of massage can be effective for reducing pain and improving mobility, it is essential for the massage therapist to adjust the pressure according to the patient's pain tolerance to avoid exacerbating symptoms.

Myofascial release is a specialized technique often incorporated into massage therapy for fibromyalgia. This approach focuses on releasing tension in the fascia, the connective tissue that surrounds muscles and organs. Myofascial release involves applying gentle, sustained pressure to the fascia, helping to alleviate pain and improve flexibility. By addressing restrictions in the fascia, this technique can help reduce the overall discomfort experienced by fibromyalgia patients.

Trigger point therapy is another technique that can be beneficial for fibromyalgia patients. Trigger points are hyperirritable spots within tight bands of muscle that can cause localized and referred pain. Trigger point therapy involves applying targeted pressure to these points to release tension and alleviate pain. This technique can be particularly effective for fibromyalgia patients who experience specific areas of muscle tightness and pain.

In addition to these techniques, massage therapists may use other methods such as hot stone massage, aromatherapy, and hydrotherapy to enhance the therapeutic effects. Hot stone massage involves the use of heated stones placed on specific areas of the body to relax muscles and improve circulation. Aromatherapy incorporates essential oils into the massage, which can have calming and pain-relieving effects. Hydrotherapy uses water in various forms, such as warm baths or whirlpools, to relax muscles and reduce pain.

Regular massage therapy sessions can provide significant benefits for fibromyalgia patients beyond pain relief. One of the key advantages is the reduction of stress and anxiety. Chronic pain and fatigue can take a toll on mental health, leading to increased levels of stress and anxiety. Massage therapy promotes relaxation and the release of endorphins, the body's natural feel-good chemicals, which can help improve mood and reduce stress. This emotional support is an essential aspect of managing fibromyalgia, as stress can exacerbate symptoms.

Improved sleep quality is another benefit of massage therapy for fibromyalgia patients. Sleep disturbances are common in fibromyalgia, often resulting in non-restorative sleep and exacerbating pain and fatigue. Massage therapy can help promote better sleep by reducing muscle tension, lowering stress levels, and encouraging relaxation. Patients who receive regular massage therapy often report improvements in their sleep patterns, feeling more rested and rejuvenated.

Cognitive Behavioral Therapy (CBT)

Cognitive Behavioral Therapy (CBT) is a well-established psychological treatment that addresses the emotional and psychological aspects of fibromyalgia. By focusing on the connection between thoughts, feelings, and behaviors, CBT helps patients develop healthier coping strategies to manage their symptoms. Given the chronic nature of fibromyalgia and its impact on daily life, CBT can be a valuable tool in reducing pain, improving mood, and enhancing overall quality of life.

CBT for fibromyalgia typically begins with a comprehensive assessment conducted by a licensed therapist or psychologist. This assessment helps identify the specific challenges and stressors the patient faces, as well as their current coping mechanisms and psychological state. The therapist and patient work together to set realistic and achievable goals for the therapy, which may include reducing pain, improving sleep, increasing activity levels, and managing stress.

One of the primary components of CBT is cognitive restructuring, which involves identifying and challenging negative thought patterns that can exacerbate fibromyalgia symptoms. Patients with fibromyalgia often experience catastrophic thinking, where they may overestimate the severity of their symptoms and underestimate their ability to cope. For example, a patient might think, "I will never be able to manage my pain, and my life will always be miserable." Cognitive restructuring helps patients recognize these negative thoughts and replace them with more balanced and realistic perspectives, such as, "While my pain is challenging, I have strategies to manage it, and I can still find joy in my life."

Another key aspect of CBT is behavioral activation, which encourages patients to engage in activities that they may have been avoiding due to pain or fear of exacerbating symptoms. Avoidance behaviors can lead to decreased physical activity, social isolation, and a lower quality of life. By gradually increasing participation in enjoyable and meaningful activities, patients can break the cycle of avoidance and inactivity. This process often involves setting small, manageable goals and gradually building up to more significant activities, fostering a sense of accomplishment and increasing overall activity levels.

CBT also includes relaxation techniques and stress management strategies to help patients cope with the physical and emotional stressors of fibromyalgia. Techniques such as deep breathing exercises, progressive muscle relaxation, guided imagery, and mindfulness meditation can reduce stress and promote relaxation. These practices help calm the nervous system, decrease muscle tension, and improve sleep quality, which are essential for managing fibromyalgia symptoms. Patients learn to incorporate these techniques into their daily routines, providing them with practical tools to manage stress and pain.

Acupuncture

Acupuncture, an ancient practice rooted in Traditional Chinese Medicine (TCM), is increasingly recognized as a complementary treatment for fibromyalgia. This holistic approach involves the insertion of thin, sterile needles into specific points on the body, known as acupoints, to stimulate the body's natural healing processes. For individuals with fibromyalgia, acupuncture can help alleviate pain, reduce muscle stiffness, and promote overall well-being.

The fundamental principle behind acupuncture is the concept of Qi (pronounced "chee"), which is considered the vital life force that flows through the body along pathways known as meridians. According to TCM, illness and pain occur when the flow of Qi is disrupted or imbalanced. Acupuncture aims to restore the balance and flow of Qi by stimulating specific acupoints, thereby promoting health and relieving symptoms.

Acupuncture treatment for fibromyalgia typically begins with a comprehensive assessment by a licensed acupuncturist. This assessment includes a detailed discussion of the patient's medical history, symptoms, lifestyle, and overall health. The acupuncturist may also conduct a physical examination, which can include palpating specific areas of the body to identify tenderness or tension. Based on this assessment, the acupuncturist develops a personalized treatment plan tailored to the patient's unique needs.

During an acupuncture session, the patient lies comfortably on a treatment table while the acupuncturist inserts thin needles into selected acupoints. The number and placement of needles depend on the patient's symptoms and the acupuncturist's assessment. Common acupoints used for fibromyalgia include those located on the back, neck, shoulders, and limbs. The insertion of the needles is generally painless, although patients may feel a slight tingling or dull ache at the site. The needles are typically left in place for 20 to 40 minutes, during which the patient can relax in a calm, soothing environment.

Acupuncture is believed to work through several mechanisms. One key mechanism is the stimulation of the nervous system, which leads to the release of endorphins and other neurotransmitters that help reduce pain and promote relaxation. Endorphins are the body's natural painkillers, and their increased release can help alleviate the chronic pain associated with fibromyalgia. Additionally, acupuncture can influence the autonomic nervous system, promoting a state of relaxation and reducing stress, which are crucial for managing fibromyalgia symptoms.

Another proposed mechanism is the improvement of blood circulation. By stimulating specific acupoints, acupuncture can enhance blood flow to affected areas, providing essential nutrients and oxygen to tissues and promoting the removal of metabolic waste products. Improved circulation can help reduce muscle stiffness and pain, contributing to overall symptom relief.

Acupuncture also addresses the mind-body connection, which is particularly relevant for fibromyalgia patients who often experience both physical and emotional symptoms. The relaxation and stress-reducing effects of acupuncture can help improve mood, reduce anxiety, and enhance sleep quality. Many fibromyalgia patients report feeling more relaxed and rejuvenated after acupuncture sessions, with improvements in their overall sense of well-being.

Tai Chi and Yoga

Tai Chi and yoga are two mind-body practices that have gained recognition for their ability to help manage the symptoms of fibromyalgia. Both practices combine physical movement, meditation, and breathing exercises to promote relaxation, improve flexibility, and enhance overall well-being. For individuals with fibromyalgia, incorporating Tai Chi and yoga into their treatment regimen can lead to significant improvements in pain, sleep, and quality of life.

Tai Chi, an ancient Chinese martial art, is characterized by slow, deliberate movements, deep breathing, and a meditative focus. Often described as "meditation in motion," Tai Chi emphasizes the cultivation of Qi (life energy) through gentle, flowing movements that enhance balance, flexibility, and strength. For fibromyalgia patients, Tai Chi offers a low-impact exercise option that can be adapted to suit various fitness levels and physical limitations.

The practice of Tai Chi involves a series of postures or forms that are performed in a continuous, smooth flow. These movements are designed to improve the body's alignment, enhance coordination, and promote relaxation. Each form transitions seamlessly into the next, creating a rhythmic and calming exercise routine. Tai Chi sessions typically begin with warm-up exercises to loosen the muscles and joints, followed by the practice of specific forms and ending with cool-down exercises to relax the body.

Yoga, with its origins in ancient India, is a holistic practice that combines physical postures (asanas), breathing techniques (pranayama), and meditation. Yoga aims to harmonize the body, mind, and spirit, promoting overall health and well-being. For fibromyalgia patients, yoga offers a versatile and adaptable form of exercise that can be tailored to meet individual needs and capabilities.

The physical postures of yoga range from gentle stretches to more challenging poses, each designed to enhance strength, flexibility, and balance. Yoga sessions typically begin with a warm-up to prepare the body, followed by a series of postures and ending with relaxation and meditation. There are various styles of yoga, each with its own focus and intensity. For fibromyalgia patients, styles such as Hatha yoga, restorative yoga, and gentle yoga are particularly beneficial as they emphasize slow, mindful movements and deep relaxation.

Occupational Therapy

Occupational therapy (OT) is a vital component of a comprehensive fibromyalgia treatment plan, aimed at helping patients manage their daily activities and improve their quality of life. Occupational therapists are healthcare professionals who specialize in assisting individuals with physical, mental, or cognitive impairments to achieve greater independence and functionality. For fibromyalgia patients, OT focuses on teaching strategies to manage pain, reduce fatigue, and optimize energy use in everyday tasks.

The first step in occupational therapy is a thorough assessment of the patient's functional abilities, limitations, and daily routines. The occupational therapist conducts interviews and evaluations to understand the specific challenges the patient faces in their personal, professional, and social life. This assessment helps the therapist develop a personalized treatment plan tailored to the patient's unique needs and goals.

One of the primary goals of occupational therapy for fibromyalgia patients is pain management. Therapists teach patients various techniques to alleviate pain and prevent exacerbation of symptoms during daily activities. These techniques may include ergonomic adjustments, such as proper body mechanics and posture, to minimize strain on muscles and joints. For example, learning how to lift objects correctly, adjust workstations, and use supportive seating can significantly reduce pain and discomfort.

Energy conservation is another crucial aspect of OT for fibromyalgia. Patients often struggle with persistent fatigue, which can make even simple tasks exhausting. Occupational therapists work with patients to develop energy-saving strategies, such as pacing, planning, and prioritizing activities. Pacing involves breaking tasks into smaller, manageable steps and taking regular breaks to avoid overexertion. Planning helps patients organize their day to include rest periods and balance high-energy and low-energy activities. Prioritizing ensures that the most important tasks are completed when the patient has the most energy.

Adaptive equipment and assistive devices can also play a significant role in reducing the physical demands of daily tasks. Occupational therapists may recommend tools such as jar openers, reachers, grab bars, and shower chairs to make activities easier and safer. These devices help patients maintain independence and reduce the risk of injury or fatigue. Additionally, therapists may provide training on how to use these tools effectively and integrate them into daily routines.

Stress management and relaxation techniques are integral parts of occupational therapy for fibromyalgia. Chronic pain and fatigue can lead to increased stress and anxiety, which in turn can exacerbate fibromyalgia symptoms. Occupational therapists teach patients various relaxation methods, such as deep breathing exercises, progressive muscle relaxation, and mindfulness meditation. These techniques help calm the nervous system, reduce muscle tension, and promote a sense of well-being.

Support Groups and Counseling

Living with fibromyalgia can be an isolating experience, as the chronic pain and fatigue associated with the condition often limit social interactions and participation in activities. Support groups and counseling offer essential emotional and psychological support, helping patients cope with the challenges of fibromyalgia and improving their overall quality of life. These resources provide a sense of community, understanding, and shared experience, which can be invaluable for those managing a chronic illness.

Support groups for fibromyalgia patients bring together individuals who share similar experiences, creating a space for mutual support and encouragement. These groups can be found in various formats, including in-person meetings, online forums, and social media communities. Participating in a support group helps reduce feelings of isolation and loneliness by connecting individuals with others who understand their struggles. Sharing personal stories and experiences can validate one's feelings and foster a sense of belonging. Additionally, support groups can be a valuable source of practical advice and information. Members often share tips on managing symptoms, navigating healthcare systems, and finding effective treatments. This exchange of knowledge can empower patients to take control of their condition and explore new strategies for symptom management. Support groups also offer emotional benefits by providing a safe space for expressing feelings and frustrations. Chronic pain and fatigue can lead to emotional distress, including depression and anxiety. Talking openly about these emotions with others who can relate can be therapeutic and help alleviate the emotional burden of fibromyalgia.

Counseling provides personalized emotional and psychological support tailored to the individual's needs. Licensed therapists, such as psychologists, clinical social workers, and counselors, work with fibromyalgia patients to address the mental health aspects of living with a chronic illness. Counseling helps address the emotional and psychological impact of living with a chronic condition, reducing symptoms of depression and anxiety. Therapy can improve stress management, which is crucial for fibromyalgia patients, as stress can exacerbate physical symptoms. By developing healthier coping mechanisms, patients can enhance their resilience and overall well-being. Counseling provides several benefits for fibromyalgia patients. It helps patients set realistic goals, maintain a positive outlook, and stay motivated in their treatment journey. Therapy can also improve patients' ability to manage their condition proactively. Therapists can teach patients techniques for pain management, relaxation, and improving sleep quality.

Participating in support groups and counseling can provide significant emotional and psychological benefits. By connecting with others who understand their experiences and working with skilled therapists, patients can reduce feelings of isolation, improve their mental health, and enhance their overall quality of life. Incorporating these supportive resources into a comprehensive fibromyalgia treatment plan can help patients navigate the challenges of living with chronic pain and achieve better symptom management and emotional well-being.

CHAPTER 6: SELF-HELP TECHNIQUES

In addition to medical treatments, various self-help strategies can empower fibromyalgia patients to manage their symptoms more effectively and improve their overall quality of life. These practical techniques include diet, sleep, exercise, stress management, and maintaining a symptom tracking journal.

Diet

Diet plays a crucial role in managing fibromyalgia symptoms and overall health. While there is no one-size-fits-all diet specifically designed for fibromyalgia, making informed dietary choices can significantly impact symptom management. A balanced diet rich in essential nutrients can help reduce inflammation, boost energy levels, and support the body's overall function.

A diet rich in fruits, vegetables, lean proteins, whole grains, and healthy fats provides the necessary nutrients to support the body and reduce fatigue. Fruits and vegetables are packed with vitamins, minerals, and antioxidants, which help combat inflammation and oxidative stress. Leafy greens like spinach, kale, and Swiss chard, as well as colorful vegetables like bell peppers, tomatoes, and carrots, are excellent choices. Fruits such as berries, apples, and citrus fruits are also beneficial due to their high antioxidant content.

Incorporating lean proteins into your diet is essential for muscle repair and maintenance. Sources of lean protein include poultry, fish, beans, lentils, and tofu. Fish, particularly fatty fish like salmon, mackerel, and sardines, are rich in omega-3 fatty acids, which have powerful anti-inflammatory properties. Omega-3 fatty acids can help reduce inflammation and pain, making them particularly beneficial for fibromyalgia patients. Plant-based protein sources, such as legumes, nuts, and seeds, also provide valuable nutrients and healthy fats.

Whole grains, such as brown rice, quinoa, oats, and whole wheat, are excellent sources of complex carbohydrates that provide sustained energy. These grains are rich in fiber, which aids digestion and helps maintain stable blood sugar levels. Stable blood sugar levels are crucial for managing energy levels and preventing the fatigue commonly associated with fibromyalgia. Additionally, whole grains contain essential vitamins and minerals, such as B vitamins, which support energy production and overall health.

Healthy fats are an important part of a balanced diet. In addition to omega-3 fatty acids, other sources of healthy fats include avocados, nuts, seeds, and olive oil. These fats support brain function, reduce inflammation, and provide a source of long-lasting energy. It is important to choose healthy fats over unhealthy fats, such as trans fats and saturated fats, which can contribute to inflammation and negatively impact health.

Hydration is another critical aspect of diet for fibromyalgia management. Drinking plenty of water throughout the day helps maintain energy levels, supports digestion, and aids in the elimination of toxins from the body. Dehydration can exacerbate fatigue and muscle pain, so it is essential to stay well-hydrated. Aim to drink at least eight glasses of water daily, and adjust your intake based on activity levels and climate. Limiting caffeinated and sugary drinks is also advisable, as they can contribute to dehydration and energy crashes.

Some fibromyalgia patients find that certain foods can trigger or worsen their symptoms. Common culprits include processed foods, refined sugars, caffeine, and artificial additives. Processed foods often contain high levels of unhealthy fats, sugars, and preservatives, which can contribute to inflammation and exacerbate symptoms. Refined sugars can cause blood sugar spikes and crashes, leading to fluctuations in energy levels. Caffeine, while it may provide a temporary energy boost, can interfere with sleep and increase anxiety, both of which can worsen fibromyalgia symptoms. Artificial additives, such as artificial sweeteners and flavor enhancers, may also trigger symptoms in some individuals.

Keeping a food diary can be an effective way to identify potential trigger foods. By tracking what you eat and noting any resulting symptoms, you can pinpoint foods that may be contributing to your discomfort. Once identified, eliminating or reducing these foods from your diet can help alleviate symptoms and improve overall well-being.

In addition to avoiding trigger foods, some patients find relief through specific dietary approaches. For example, an anti-inflammatory diet focuses on foods that reduce inflammation, such as fruits, vegetables, whole grains, lean proteins, and healthy fats. This type of diet minimizes foods that can cause inflammation, such as refined sugars, unhealthy fats, and processed foods. Another approach is the Mediterranean diet, which emphasizes fruits, vegetables, whole grains, fish, nuts, and olive oil, and has been shown to reduce inflammation and improve overall health.

For some fibromyalgia patients, food sensitivities or allergies may play a role in symptom management. Common food sensitivities include gluten, dairy, and certain additives. If you suspect that food sensitivities are affecting your symptoms, consider working with a healthcare provider or registered dietitian to identify and eliminate potential allergens from your diet. An elimination diet, where you remove suspected foods and then gradually reintroduce them while monitoring symptoms, can be a useful tool in identifying food sensitivities.

Sleep

Quality sleep is vital for managing fibromyalgia, as poor sleep can exacerbate pain and fatigue, leading to a vicious cycle of worsening symptoms. Establishing good sleep hygiene practices can significantly improve sleep quality and help manage symptoms more effectively. One of the first steps in improving sleep is to maintain a regular sleep schedule. Going to bed and waking up at the same time every day, even on weekends, helps regulate the body's internal clock and can improve overall sleep patterns. Consistency reinforces the body's natural sleep-wake cycle, making it easier to fall asleep and wake up feeling refreshed.

Creating a comfortable sleep environment is also crucial. The bedroom should be a sanctuary for sleep, free from distractions and conducive to relaxation. Ensure the room is cool, quiet, and dark. Using blackout curtains or a sleep mask can help block out light, while earplugs or a white noise machine can minimize disruptive sounds. Investing in a supportive mattress and pillows can make a significant difference in sleep quality. A mattress that provides adequate support and comfort tailored to your body type and sleeping position can help reduce pain and improve sleep.

Establishing a relaxing bedtime routine can signal to your body that it's time to wind down. Engaging in calming activities before bed can help transition from wakefulness to sleepiness. Consider incorporating activities such as reading a book, taking a warm bath, or practicing gentle stretching exercises. These activities can promote relaxation and prepare you for sleep. Avoiding stimulating activities before bed, such as watching TV, using electronic devices, or engaging in intense exercise, is also important. The blue light emitted by screens can interfere with the production of the sleep hormone melatonin, making it harder to fall asleep. Instead, opt for activities that promote relaxation and reduce stress.

Diet and sleep are closely linked, and certain dietary habits can impact sleep quality. Limiting the intake of caffeine and alcohol, especially in the evening, can help prevent sleep disturbances. Caffeine is a stimulant that can interfere with falling asleep, while alcohol can disrupt the sleep cycle, leading to fragmented and less restful sleep. Additionally, avoiding large meals and heavy, rich foods before bedtime can prevent discomfort and indigestion that might interfere with sleep. Opting for a light, healthy snack if you are hungry can help you sleep better.

Regular physical activity can also contribute to better sleep, although the timing of exercise is important. Engaging in regular exercise can help reduce stress, improve mood, and promote restful sleep. However, vigorous exercise too close to bedtime can be stimulating and may make it harder to fall asleep. Aim to complete any intense workouts at least a few hours before bedtime, while gentle exercises like yoga or stretching can be part of your pre-sleep routine.

Stress and anxiety are common culprits of sleep disturbances, particularly for individuals with fibromyalgia. Developing effective stress management techniques can improve sleep quality. Techniques such as mindfulness meditation, deep breathing exercises, progressive muscle relaxation, and guided imagery can help calm the mind and prepare the body for sleep. These practices can be incorporated into your bedtime routine or used throughout the day to manage stress.

Sleep disorders, such as insomnia, sleep apnea, and restless legs syndrome, are common among fibromyalgia patients and can significantly impact sleep quality. If you suspect that a sleep disorder is contributing to your sleep problems, it is important to seek professional evaluation and treatment. A sleep specialist can conduct assessments, such as a sleep study, to diagnose any underlying sleep disorders and recommend appropriate treatments. Treatments may include continuous positive airway pressure (CPAP) therapy for sleep apnea, medications, or other interventions tailored to your specific needs.

In addition to these strategies, cognitive-behavioral therapy for insomnia (CBT-I) can be an effective treatment for improving sleep quality. CBT-I is a structured program that helps individuals identify and change thoughts and behaviors that negatively impact sleep. By addressing these underlying issues, CBT-I can help improve sleep patterns and overall sleep quality. Working with a trained therapist, patients can learn techniques to manage racing thoughts, reduce nighttime awakenings, and establish healthier sleep habits.

Exercise

Regular exercise is one of the most effective ways to manage fibromyalgia symptoms, offering numerous benefits such as pain reduction, improved sleep, enhanced mood, and increased energy levels. However, for individuals with fibromyalgia, finding the right balance in an exercise routine can be challenging due to the condition's characteristic pain and fatigue. It is essential to approach exercise with caution, starting slowly and gradually increasing the intensity and duration to avoid overexertion and symptom flare-ups.

Low-impact aerobic exercises are highly recommended for fibromyalgia patients as they provide cardiovascular benefits without putting excessive strain on the joints and muscles. Activities such as walking, swimming, and cycling are excellent options. Walking is a simple and accessible form of exercise that can be easily incorporated into daily routines. It helps improve cardiovascular health, boosts mood, and can be adjusted in intensity and duration based on individual fitness levels. Swimming and water aerobics are particularly beneficial due to the buoyancy provided by water, which reduces the stress on joints and allows for gentle, full-body workouts. Cycling, whether on a stationary bike or outdoors, offers a low-impact way to enhance cardiovascular fitness and build leg strength.

Strength training is another important component of a well-rounded exercise program for fibromyalgia patients. Building muscle strength can help support joints, improve posture, and enhance overall physical function. It is crucial to start with light weights or resistance bands and focus on proper form to prevent injury. Exercises such as seated leg presses, bicep curls, and shoulder presses can be performed using resistance bands or light dumbbells. Gradually increasing the resistance as strength improves can help patients gain confidence and maintain progress without overloading the muscles.

Flexibility and stretching exercises are essential for reducing muscle stiffness and improving range of motion. Gentle stretching can help alleviate muscle tension and prevent the formation of painful trigger points. Practices such as yoga and Tai Chi combine stretching with relaxation techniques, making them particularly beneficial for fibromyalgia patients. Yoga involves a series of postures that promote flexibility, strength, and balance. It also incorporates deep breathing and mindfulness, which can help reduce stress and enhance overall well-being. Tai Chi, with its slow, deliberate movements and focus on breath control, improves flexibility and balance while promoting relaxation and mental clarity.

Regular, consistent exercise is more beneficial for fibromyalgia patients than sporadic, intense workouts. Aim for at least 20-30 minutes of moderate exercise on most days of the week. It is important to listen to your body and adjust your routine based on your energy levels and symptoms. Pacing is a critical strategy to avoid overexertion and flare-ups. Breaking exercise into shorter, manageable sessions throughout the day can make it easier to stay active without overwhelming the body. For example, three 10-minute walks can be as effective as one 30-minute session and may be more tolerable for individuals with fibromyalgia.

Warm-up and cool-down periods are essential components of any exercise routine, particularly for those with fibromyalgia. Warming up with gentle movements such as light walking or stretching prepares the muscles and joints for more strenuous activity and reduces the risk of injury. Cooling down with slow, gentle stretches helps to relax the muscles and gradually lower the heart rate, promoting recovery and reducing post-exercise soreness.

Hydration and nutrition also play vital roles in supporting an exercise regimen. Staying well-hydrated before, during, and after exercise helps maintain energy levels and prevent muscle cramps. Eating a balanced diet rich in nutrients supports overall health and provides the necessary fuel for physical activity. Consuming a small, nutritious snack, such as a piece of fruit or a handful of nuts, before exercise can provide an energy boost and enhance performance.

In addition to physical benefits, exercise offers significant psychological advantages. Engaging in regular physical activity can help reduce symptoms of depression and anxiety, which are common comorbidities in fibromyalgia patients. Exercise stimulates the release of endorphins, the body's natural mood elevators, and can provide a sense of accomplishment and empowerment. Group exercise classes, such as yoga or water aerobics, can offer social interaction and support, further enhancing mental well-being.

For those new to exercise or uncertain about how to begin, working with a physical therapist or a certified fitness trainer with experience in fibromyalgia can provide personalized guidance and support. These professionals can help design a safe and effective exercise program tailored to individual needs and limitations. They can also provide education on proper techniques and adjustments to ensure that exercises are performed correctly and safely.

Stress Management

Managing stress is a critical aspect of controlling fibromyalgia symptoms, as stress can significantly exacerbate pain, fatigue, and other symptoms. Incorporating effective stress management techniques into daily routines can help reduce overall stress levels and improve the ability to cope with fibromyalgia. Given the chronic nature of the condition, developing a comprehensive approach to stress management can lead to better symptom control and enhanced quality of life.

One of the most effective stress management techniques is meditation. Meditation involves focusing the mind and eliminating distractions to achieve a state of deep relaxation and mental clarity. There are various forms of meditation, including mindfulness meditation, guided meditation, and transcendental meditation.

Mindfulness meditation encourages awareness of the present moment without judgment, helping individuals develop a greater sense of acceptance and peace. Guided meditation involves listening to a recorded guide that leads the participant through a series of calming visualizations and affirmations. Regular practice of meditation can help calm the mind, reduce stress, and promote relaxation, making it an invaluable tool for managing fibromyalgia symptoms.

Mindfulness practices extend beyond formal meditation sessions and can be integrated into daily activities. Mindfulness involves paying attention to the present moment with a sense of curiosity and acceptance. Simple mindfulness exercises, such as mindful breathing, mindful eating, or mindful walking, can help reduce stress and improve mental clarity. For example, mindful breathing involves focusing on the breath, noticing the sensation of air entering and leaving the body, and gently bringing the mind back to the breath whenever it wanders. This practice can be done anywhere and at any time, making it a versatile tool for managing stress.

Relaxation techniques are also essential for stress management in fibromyalgia patients. Deep breathing exercises, progressive muscle relaxation, and guided imagery are effective methods for promoting relaxation and reducing muscle tension. Deep breathing exercises involve taking slow, deep breaths, filling the lungs fully, and then exhaling slowly. This practice helps activate the body's relaxation response and can be particularly helpful during moments of acute stress or pain. Progressive muscle relaxation involves tensing and then relaxing different muscle groups in the body, starting from the feet and working up to the head. This technique can help release physical tension and promote a sense of calm. Guided imagery involves visualizing a peaceful and calming scene, such as a beach or a forest, and focusing on the sensory details of that scene. This practice can help distract the mind from pain and stress, promoting relaxation and mental clarity.

Physical activity, while discussed as a separate topic, is also a vital component of stress management. Regular exercise helps reduce stress hormones like cortisol and promotes the release of endorphins, which are natural mood elevators. Activities such as yoga and Tai Chi are particularly beneficial as they combine physical movement with mindfulness and breathing techniques, providing a holistic approach to stress reduction. Engaging in enjoyable physical activities can also serve as a healthy distraction from pain and stress.

Social support is another crucial element of stress management. Connecting with others who understand the challenges of living with fibromyalgia can provide emotional support and reduce feelings of isolation. Participating in support groups, whether in-person or online, allows individuals to share their experiences, learn from others, and receive encouragement. Friends, family members, and healthcare providers can also be valuable sources of support. Building a strong support network can help patients feel more understood and less alone in their journey.

Creating a structured daily routine can also help manage stress. Establishing regular times for meals, exercise, relaxation, and sleep can create a sense of predictability and stability, which can be comforting and reduce stress. Planning and prioritizing activities can help manage energy levels and prevent overexertion. Breaking tasks into smaller, manageable steps and taking regular breaks can make daily activities more manageable and less overwhelming.

Symptom Tracking Journal

Maintaining a symptom tracking journal can be an invaluable tool for managing fibromyalgia. By keeping a detailed record of your symptoms, you can identify patterns, triggers, and effective strategies for relief. This proactive approach not only helps you gain a deeper understanding of your condition but also provides essential information that can guide treatment decisions and enhance communication with healthcare providers.

A symptom tracking journal involves recording your symptoms daily, noting their severity, duration, and any potential triggers. This detailed documentation helps capture the nuances of fibromyalgia, which can vary greatly from day to day. By consistently tracking your symptoms, you create a comprehensive picture of your health, enabling you to see trends and correlations that may not be immediately apparent.

Start by noting the date and time of each entry, along with a description of your symptoms. Include details such as the type of pain you are experiencing (e.g., sharp, dull, throbbing), its location, and intensity. Using a pain scale from 1 to 10 can help quantify the severity of your symptoms. Additionally, record other symptoms such as fatigue, sleep disturbances, cognitive difficulties, stiffness, and mood changes. This holistic approach ensures that all aspects of your condition are documented.

In your journal, also include information about your daily activities, diet, sleep patterns, exercise routines, stress levels, and any treatments or medications you used. This comprehensive approach helps identify potential triggers and lifestyle factors that influence your symptoms. For example, you might discover that certain foods exacerbate your pain, or that a particular type of exercise helps alleviate stiffness. Documenting your activities and their impact on your symptoms can provide valuable insights into what helps or hinders your condition.

Tracking your diet is particularly important, as certain foods may trigger symptoms or affect your overall well-being. Record what you eat and drink throughout the day, noting any reactions you experience. Pay attention to potential dietary triggers such as processed foods, sugar, caffeine, and artificial additives. Over time, you may notice patterns that can guide you in making dietary adjustments to reduce symptom flare-ups.

Sleep quality is another crucial aspect to monitor in your symptom tracking journal. Record the number of hours you sleep each night, the quality of your sleep, and any difficulties you experience, such as trouble falling asleep, frequent awakenings, or unrefreshing sleep. Note any sleep hygiene practices you follow, such as maintaining a regular sleep schedule, creating a comfortable sleep environment, and avoiding stimulants before bed. Tracking your sleep can help identify factors that contribute to poor sleep quality and guide you in making improvements to enhance restorative sleep.

Exercise and physical activity are important components of fibromyalgia management, and documenting your routines can help you understand their impact on your symptoms. Record the type, duration, and intensity of your exercise, as well as how you feel before, during, and after the activity. This information can help you determine the most beneficial types of exercise and the appropriate intensity level for your condition. It can also highlight the importance of pacing and rest periods to avoid overexertion and flare-ups.

Stress is a significant factor in fibromyalgia, and tracking your stress levels and stress management techniques can provide valuable insights. Document your stress levels throughout the day and any stressors you encounter. Note the techniques you use to manage stress, such as meditation, deep breathing, or journaling, and their effectiveness in reducing stress and improving symptoms. This information can help you refine your stress management strategies and develop a more effective approach to coping with stress.

Reviewing your journal regularly can help you identify patterns and correlations between your activities and symptoms. For example, you might notice that certain foods or activities consistently trigger symptoms, or that specific treatments provide relief. This information can guide you in making informed adjustments to your lifestyle and treatment plan. Additionally, sharing your symptom tracking journal with your healthcare providers can provide valuable insights and help them better understand your condition. It can also aid in developing a more personalized and effective treatment plan, as your doctor can see firsthand how different factors affect your symptoms.

CHAPTER 7: SUPPLEMENTS AND HERBAL REMEDIES

For many individuals with fibromyalgia, conventional treatments alone may not provide complete relief from symptoms. Supplements and herbal remedies can offer additional support, potentially helping to manage pain, fatigue, and other related symptoms. This chapter explores various supplements and herbal remedies that have been used to treat fibromyalgia symptoms, providing insights into their potential benefits, how they work, and considerations for their use.

Supplements

Vitamin D

Vitamin D plays a crucial role in bone health, immune function, and muscle function. Deficiency in vitamin D has been linked to increased pain sensitivity and musculoskeletal pain, which are common in fibromyalgia patients. Supplementing with vitamin D may help reduce pain and improve overall well-being. It is important to have your vitamin D levels checked by a healthcare provider before starting supplementation, as excessive intake can lead to toxicity.

Magnesium

Magnesium is essential for muscle and nerve function, and many people with fibromyalgia have been found to have lower levels of this mineral. Magnesium supplements can help reduce muscle cramps, improve sleep quality, and alleviate pain. Magnesium citrate and magnesium glycinate are popular forms of supplementation due to their high bioavailability and minimal gastrointestinal side effects.

Omega-3 Fatty Acids

Omega-3 fatty acids, found in fish oil supplements, have potent anti-inflammatory properties. Chronic inflammation is believed to play a role in fibromyalgia, and omega-3 supplementation can help reduce inflammation and pain. Additionally, omega-3s support heart health and cognitive function. It is recommended to choose high-quality fish oil supplements that are free from contaminants such as mercury.

Coenzyme Q10 (CoQ10)

CoQ10 is a powerful antioxidant that plays a vital role in energy production within cells. Some studies have suggested that CoQ10 levels are lower in fibromyalgia patients, which may contribute to fatigue and muscle pain. Supplementing with CoQ10 can help improve energy levels, reduce fatigue, and enhance overall mitochondrial function.

Melatonin

Sleep disturbances are a significant issue for many fibromyalgia patients, and melatonin, a natural hormone that regulates sleep-wake cycles, can be beneficial. Melatonin supplements can help improve sleep quality and duration, making it easier for patients to achieve restorative sleep. It is best to start with a low dose and gradually increase as needed, under the guidance of a healthcare provider.

5-HTP (5-Hydroxytryptophan)

5-HTP is a naturally occurring amino acid that is a precursor to serotonin, a neurotransmitter that affects mood, sleep, and pain perception. Low levels of serotonin are often associated with fibromyalgia. Supplementing with 5-HTP can help increase serotonin levels, potentially improving mood, reducing pain, and enhancing sleep quality. However, it is essential to consult with a healthcare provider before using 5-HTP, especially if you are taking antidepressants, as it can interact with these medications.

Herbal Remedies

Turmeric (Curcuma longa)

Turmeric is a spice known for its anti-inflammatory and antioxidant properties, primarily due to its active component, curcumin. Curcumin can help reduce inflammation and oxidative stress, which are thought to contribute to fibromyalgia symptoms. Incorporating turmeric into the diet or taking curcumin supplements can provide relief from pain and improve overall health. It is important to choose curcumin supplements with enhanced bioavailability, such as those combined with black pepper extract (piperine).

Ginger (Zingiber officinale)

Ginger has long been used for its anti-inflammatory and analgesic properties. It can help reduce muscle pain and stiffness associated with fibromyalgia. Ginger can be consumed in various forms, including fresh ginger root, ginger tea, or supplements. It also has the added benefit of aiding digestion and reducing nausea, which can be beneficial for those with fibromyalgia-related gastrointestinal issues.

St. John's Wort (Hypericum perforatum)

St. John's Wort is an herbal remedy commonly used to treat mild to moderate depression. It works by increasing levels of serotonin, dopamine, and norepinephrine in the brain, which can improve mood and alleviate some fibromyalgia symptoms. However, St. John's Wort can interact with several medications, including antidepressants, birth control pills, and blood thinners. It is crucial to consult with a healthcare provider before using this herb.

Valerian Root (Valeriana officinalis)

Valerian root is an herbal remedy often used to promote relaxation and improve sleep quality. Its sedative properties can help reduce anxiety and insomnia, which are common in fibromyalgia patients. Valerian root can be consumed as a tea, tincture, or supplement. It is important to use valerian root under the guidance of a healthcare provider, especially if you are taking other medications or have liver issues.

Boswellia (Boswellia serrata)

Boswellia, also known as Indian frankincense, is an herbal remedy with strong anti-inflammatory properties. It can help reduce inflammation and pain associated with fibromyalgia. Boswellia supplements are available in various forms, including capsules and tablets. When choosing a supplement, look for products standardized to contain a high percentage of boswellic acids, the active components responsible for its therapeutic effects.

Ashwagandha (Withania somnifera)

Ashwagandha is an adaptogenic herb that helps the body adapt to stress and supports overall well-being. It has been shown to reduce stress and anxiety, improve sleep quality, and boost energy levels. These benefits make ashwagandha a valuable addition to a fibromyalgia management plan. Ashwagandha can be taken as a powder, capsule, or tincture.

Considerations for Use

When considering supplements and herbal remedies, it is essential to consult with a healthcare provider to ensure they are safe and appropriate for your specific condition. Some supplements and herbs can interact with medications or have contraindications for certain health conditions. Additionally, the quality and potency of supplements and herbal products can vary widely, so it is important to choose reputable brands and products that have been tested for purity and efficacy.

Starting with a low dose and gradually increasing as needed can help minimize the risk of side effects. It is also important to monitor your symptoms and any changes in your condition while using supplements and herbal remedies. Keeping a symptom tracking journal can help you identify which products are effective and how they impact your overall well-being.

CHAPTER 8: LIVING WITH FIBROMYALGIA

Living with fibromyalgia can present numerous challenges, but with the right strategies and support, it is possible to maintain a good quality of life. This chapter provides practical advice and coping mechanisms to help manage the impacts of fibromyalgia on various aspects of life, including work, school, home life, and social interactions. By adopting a proactive approach and making thoughtful adjustments, individuals with fibromyalgia can lead fulfilling and productive lives.

Managing Work Life

Managing work life with fibromyalgia can be particularly challenging due to the condition's fluctuating nature, characterized by periods of severe pain and fatigue. However, with strategic planning, open communication, and the right accommodations, it is possible to maintain a productive and satisfying work life. The key lies in understanding your rights, advocating for necessary adjustments, and implementing effective strategies to manage your symptoms while fulfilling your job responsibilities.

Open communication with your employer is crucial when it comes to managing fibromyalgia at work. It is important to have an honest conversation with your supervisor or human resources department about your condition and how it affects your daily functioning. Explain the nature of fibromyalgia, the unpredictability of symptom flare-ups, and the specific challenges you face. Being transparent about your needs can pave the way for a more supportive work environment and help your employer understand the importance of making reasonable accommodations.

Several accommodations can be beneficial for employees with fibromyalgia. Flexible work hours can be particularly helpful, allowing you to adjust your schedule based on your energy levels and symptom severity. For instance, starting the workday later or taking extended breaks can provide the necessary rest to manage fatigue. Telecommuting or working from home, even on a part-time basis, can also be a valuable option, reducing the physical strain of commuting and allowing for a more comfortable work environment.

Ergonomic adjustments to your workstation can make a significant difference in minimizing physical discomfort. Investing in a supportive chair that promotes good posture, ensuring your computer screen is at eye level, and using a keyboard and mouse that reduce strain on your wrists can help alleviate pain and prevent exacerbation of symptoms. If your job involves standing for long periods, using a cushioned mat and wearing supportive footwear can reduce strain on your legs and back.

Pacing and energy management are essential strategies for maintaining productivity while managing fibromyalgia symptoms. Break tasks into smaller, manageable steps and prioritize high-priority items when your energy levels are at their peak. Scheduling regular breaks throughout the day to rest and stretch can prevent overexertion and reduce muscle stiffness. Using tools and technology to streamline tasks can also help conserve energy and improve efficiency. For example, using voice recognition software to dictate emails or documents can reduce the physical strain of typing.

Stress management is another critical aspect of maintaining work life with fibromyalgia. Chronic stress can exacerbate fibromyalgia symptoms, making it essential to incorporate stress reduction techniques into your daily routine. Practicing deep breathing exercises, mindfulness, or brief meditation sessions during breaks can help calm your mind and reduce stress levels. Additionally, creating a quiet and organized workspace can minimize distractions and promote a sense of calm.

Advocating for your rights in the workplace is also important. The Americans with Disabilities Act (ADA) provides protections for individuals with disabilities, including those with fibromyalgia. Under the ADA, employers are required to provide reasonable accommodations to enable employees with disabilities to perform their job functions. Familiarizing yourself with your rights under the ADA can empower you to request the necessary accommodations and ensure that your needs are met.

Several advocacy groups and networks are dedicated to supporting individuals with fibromyalgia and advocating for their rights in the workplace. Organizations such as the National Fibromyalgia Association (NFA) and the Fibromyalgia Network provide resources, support, and advocacy for people living with fibromyalgia. These organizations offer information on workplace accommodations, legal rights, and strategies for managing fibromyalgia in a professional setting. Joining a fibromyalgia support group, either in-person or online, can also provide valuable advice and encouragement from others who understand the challenges of managing work life with fibromyalgia.

In addition to seeking accommodations and support, it is important to listen to your body and adjust your work habits as needed. Recognizing your limits and taking proactive steps to manage your symptoms can prevent burnout and improve your overall well-being. If you experience a symptom flare-up, do not hesitate to communicate with your employer and take the necessary time off to recover. Using sick leave or short-term disability benefits can provide the needed respite to manage severe symptoms and prevent long-term health complications.

Maintaining a healthy work-life balance is crucial for managing fibromyalgia effectively. Ensuring that you have time for self-care, relaxation, and activities that bring you joy outside of work can improve your overall quality of life. Engaging in regular physical activity, following a balanced diet, and getting adequate sleep are essential components of managing fibromyalgia and maintaining your ability to perform well at work.

Managing School Life

Managing school life with fibromyalgia can be particularly challenging due to the physical and cognitive demands of coursework, exams, and social activities. However, with strategic planning, effective communication, and the right accommodations, students with fibromyalgia can achieve academic success while managing their symptoms. This section provides detailed strategies to help students navigate their educational journey and maintain their health and well-being.

One of the first steps in managing school life with fibromyalgia is effective communication with teachers, school administrators, and, if applicable, disability services. It is essential to inform them about your condition and how it affects your daily functioning. Providing detailed information about fibromyalgia, including the unpredictability of symptom flare-ups, can help educators understand the challenges you face. Requesting a meeting with your teachers or school officials to discuss potential accommodations and support is crucial. This proactive approach can foster a supportive educational environment and ensure that your needs are met.

Accommodations can vary depending on individual needs and the educational setting, but some common adjustments may include extended deadlines for assignments and exams, modified coursework, the option to record lectures, and preferential seating to reduce physical strain. Extended deadlines can provide the necessary flexibility to manage workload without compromising academic performance. Modified coursework, such as reduced reading or alternative assignments, can help balance academic demands with health needs. Recording lectures allows students to review material at their own pace, ensuring they do not miss important information during periods of cognitive fog or fatigue. Preferential seating can help minimize physical discomfort and make it easier to access necessary resources.

Developing a structured routine is another key strategy for managing school life with fibromyalgia. Creating a consistent schedule that includes regular study sessions, breaks, and time for self-care can help balance academic responsibilities and personal well-being. Using tools like planners, calendars, or digital apps to organize assignments, exams, and other commitments can help manage time effectively. Breaking down study sessions into shorter, focused intervals with regular breaks can improve concentration and prevent fatigue. For example, the Pomodoro Technique, which involves studying for 25 minutes followed by a 5-minute break, can be particularly effective in maintaining focus and productivity.

Energy management and pacing are critical for students with fibromyalgia. It is essential to prioritize tasks and focus on completing high-priority items when your energy levels are at their peak. Scheduling more demanding activities, such as studying for exams or working on projects, during times when you feel most alert and capable can improve efficiency and reduce the risk of symptom flare-ups. Incorporating rest periods throughout the day and taking advantage of any free time to rest or engage in relaxing activities can help manage fatigue. Learning to listen to your body and recognizing signs of overexertion is crucial in preventing burnout.

Seeking support from peers, study groups, or tutoring services can provide academic assistance and emotional support. Joining a study group can enhance understanding of course material and provide a sense of camaraderie. Peers who are aware of your condition can offer encouragement and help you stay motivated.

Utilizing tutoring services can provide additional academic support and ensure you keep up with coursework during periods of increased symptoms.

Accessing disability services, if available, can provide additional resources and support. Disability services offices can help coordinate accommodations, provide advocacy, and offer tools and strategies for managing academic responsibilities. They can also assist in communicating with faculty and ensuring that accommodations are implemented effectively.

Managing Home Life

Creating a supportive home environment begins with organizing your living space to minimize physical strain and make daily tasks more manageable. Start by decluttering and arranging your home to keep frequently used items within easy reach. This reduces the need for excessive bending, stretching, or lifting, which can exacerbate pain and fatigue. For example, store kitchen essentials like utensils, pots, and pans at waist level, and use shelving units to keep items accessible without having to reach too high or low. In the bathroom, use shower caddies and wall-mounted organizers to keep toiletries within easy reach.

Utilizing assistive devices can significantly ease the burden of household chores. Tools such as jar openers, electric can openers, reachers, grab bars, and shower chairs can make tasks easier and safer. For example, a lightweight vacuum cleaner can reduce the strain of cleaning floors, while a long-handled duster can help reach high places without stretching. Investing in ergonomic tools designed to reduce physical effort can help conserve energy and prevent injury.

Pacing is a crucial strategy for managing home responsibilities. Break tasks into smaller, manageable steps and spread them throughout the day or week to avoid overexertion. Prioritize essential tasks and focus on completing high-priority items first. For instance, you might clean one room at a time or do a small load of laundry each day instead of attempting to complete all household chores in one go. Use a timer to remind yourself to take breaks, and listen to your body's signals to rest when needed. Pacing helps balance activity with rest, preventing flare-ups and maintaining a steady level of productivity.

Establishing a daily routine that includes time for self-care, relaxation, and activities you enjoy is vital for balancing responsibilities and personal well-being. Incorporate regular rest periods into your schedule to recharge and manage fatigue. Designate specific times for household chores, meals, exercise, and leisure activities. A structured routine can create a sense of predictability and stability, which can be comforting and reduce stress. Flexibility within your routine is also important, allowing you to adjust plans based on your energy levels and symptoms on any given day.

Delegating responsibilities to family members or hiring help can lighten the load and ensure that essential tasks are completed without overburdening yourself. Communicate openly with your family about your needs and limitations, and involve them in sharing household duties. For example, children can help with tidying up their rooms, setting the table, or folding laundry, while a spouse or partner can assist with more physically demanding tasks like grocery shopping or yard work. If feasible, consider hiring professional cleaning services or a personal assistant to handle specific chores.

Creating a comfortable and relaxing space within your home is essential for managing fibromyalgia symptoms. Designate a quiet area for relaxation and self-care, where you can retreat when you need to rest or engage in calming activities. This space might include a comfortable chair or bed, soft lighting, and items that bring you comfort, such as books, music, or aromatherapy diffusers. Practicing relaxation techniques such as deep breathing exercises, progressive muscle relaxation, or guided imagery in this space can help reduce stress and promote a sense of well-being.

Adapting meal preparation to accommodate your energy levels and physical limitations can make cooking more manageable. Plan meals in advance and consider batch cooking or using a slow cooker to prepare meals with minimal effort. Keep healthy, easy-to-prepare snacks on hand for times when you have low energy. Utilize kitchen gadgets like food processors, electric can openers, and lightweight cookware to reduce the physical strain of cooking. Simplifying meal preparation can help ensure you maintain a nutritious diet without overexerting yourself.

Managing Social Life

One of the first steps in managing your social life is open and honest communication with your friends and family about your condition. Educate them about fibromyalgia, explaining its symptoms and how it affects your daily life. Many people may not understand the invisible nature of the illness and the variability of its symptoms. Sharing information about your condition can foster understanding and empathy, which are essential for building supportive relationships. Let your loved ones know what you need in terms of support, whether it is physical assistance, emotional encouragement, or simply patience and understanding.

Planning social activities that accommodate your energy levels and physical limitations is crucial. Opt for activities that are less physically demanding and can be easily adjusted based on how you are feeling. For example, instead of a strenuous hike, you might suggest a leisurely walk in the park or a picnic. Quiet dinners at home, movie nights, and small gatherings can also be enjoyable without being overly taxing. Flexibility is key—choose activities that can be modified or postponed if you experience a flare-up or are feeling particularly fatigued.

Pacing is essential when it comes to social engagements. Spread out social activities to avoid overcommitting and ensure you have adequate rest between events. For example, if you have a busy weekend planned, make sure to schedule downtime before and after to recuperate. Listening to your body and recognizing your limits can help prevent overexertion and subsequent flare-ups. It's important to communicate with your friends and family about the need for pacing so they understand why you might need to leave early or take breaks during activities.

When attending social events, consider practical strategies to manage your symptoms. For example, bring a cushion or portable chair for extra comfort, wear comfortable clothing and supportive footwear, and ensure you have easy access to medications or other items that help manage your symptoms. If you're attending an event that involves a lot of standing or walking, plan ahead to take breaks and find places to sit and rest. Communicating your needs to event organizers or hosts can help ensure that accommodations are made to support your comfort and participation.

Managing stress is a crucial aspect of maintaining a social life with fibromyalgia. Social interactions can sometimes be stressful, especially if you are worried about managing symptoms in public or feeling pressure to meet social expectations. Incorporating stress management techniques into your daily routine can help reduce anxiety and improve your ability to enjoy social activities. Techniques such as mindfulness meditation, deep breathing exercises, and progressive muscle relaxation can promote relaxation and enhance your overall well-being.

Being adaptable and flexible is crucial. There may be times when you need to cancel plans or leave an event early due to a flare-up or extreme fatigue. Communicate openly with your friends and family about these possibilities so they understand that your condition can be unpredictable. Most importantly, be kind to yourself and allow yourself the grace to prioritize your health without feeling guilty.

Building a Support Network

Building a strong support network is essential for managing fibromyalgia effectively and maintaining a good quality of life. A robust support system can provide emotional encouragement, practical assistance, and a sense of community, all of which are crucial for navigating the challenges of living with a chronic condition. This section offers practical steps and resources to help you build and maintain a supportive network.

One of the first steps in building a support network is to educate your immediate family and close friends about fibromyalgia. Many people may not fully understand the condition or the impact it has on your daily life. Sharing information about fibromyalgia, including its symptoms, triggers, and the variability of its severity, can foster empathy and understanding. You can provide them with articles, books, or reliable online resources that explain the condition. Encouraging open and honest communication about your needs and limitations can help your loved ones understand how to best support you.

Joining a fibromyalgia support group is an excellent way to connect with others who share similar experiences. These groups offer a platform for sharing coping strategies, receiving encouragement, and discussing the challenges and triumphs of living with fibromyalgia. Support groups can be found both in-person and online, providing flexibility to choose the format that best suits your needs. In-person support groups are often organized by local hospitals, community centers, or fibromyalgia advocacy organizations. Websites such as the National Fibromyalgia Association (NFA) and the Fibromyalgia Network offer directories of local support groups. Online support groups and forums, such as those on Facebook or health-related websites like PatientsLikeMe, provide an accessible option for those who may have difficulty attending in-person meetings.

Building a support network extends beyond family, friends, and healthcare providers to include broader community resources. Many communities offer resources for individuals with chronic illnesses, such as adaptive exercise classes, wellness workshops, and educational seminars. Check with local community centers, hospitals, and health organizations to find out what resources are available in your area. Participating in these programs can help you stay active, learn new coping strategies, and connect with others who understand your experience.

Utilizing technology can also enhance your support network. There are numerous apps and online platforms designed to help individuals manage chronic conditions and connect with others. Apps like MyFibroTeam and CareZone offer tools for tracking symptoms, managing medications, and connecting with a community of peers. These platforms provide a convenient way to stay organized and engaged with your health management while accessing support from others with similar experiences.

To maintain a strong support network, it is essential to nurture your relationships. Regular communication with your support system, whether through phone calls, video chats, or in-person visits, can help maintain connections and provide ongoing emotional support. Expressing gratitude and appreciation for the support you receive can strengthen these relationships and encourage continued support. Being open about your needs and how your support system can help you can also foster a sense of partnership and understanding.

Self-advocacy is another important component of building a support network. Learning to advocate for your needs, whether in medical settings, at work, or in social situations, can empower you to take control of your health and well-being. This might involve requesting specific accommodations at work, seeking second opinions or additional treatments from healthcare providers, or setting boundaries in your personal relationships to protect your energy and health. Advocacy organizations often provide resources and training on self-advocacy skills, helping you become a more effective advocate for your needs.

CHAPTER 9: THE FUTURE OF FIBROMYALGIA

As our understanding of fibromyalgia continues to evolve, so too does the landscape of potential treatments and research dedicated to this complex condition. The future of fibromyalgia holds promise, with emerging therapies, innovative research, and a growing awareness that may lead to more effective management and improved quality of life for those affected by the condition. In this final chapter, we explore the exciting advancements on the horizon and highlight ongoing studies that are shaping the future of fibromyalgia treatment and care.

Emerging Treatments

The quest for more effective treatments for fibromyalgia is ongoing, with researchers exploring a variety of novel approaches. One promising area of development is the use of neuromodulation techniques. These methods involve stimulating specific areas of the nervous system to alleviate pain and improve function. Techniques such as transcranial magnetic stimulation (TMS) and transcutaneous electrical nerve stimulation (TENS) have shown potential in reducing pain and improving quality of life for fibromyalgia patients. TMS, which uses magnetic fields to stimulate nerve cells in the brain, has been studied for its effects on pain modulation and mood improvement. Similarly, TENS, which involves applying electrical currents to the skin to relieve pain, has been investigated for its potential to provide relief from fibromyalgia symptoms.

Pharmacological advancements are also being made, with new medications being developed and tested for their efficacy in treating fibromyalgia. Researchers are exploring the use of medications that target specific pathways involved in pain processing and inflammation. For example, drugs that modulate the activity of glial cells, which play a role in the immune response and inflammation in the nervous system, are being investigated for their potential to reduce pain and improve function. Additionally, cannabinoids, compounds derived from the cannabis plant, are being studied for their analgesic and anti-inflammatory properties. Preliminary research suggests that cannabinoids may help alleviate pain and improve sleep in fibromyalgia patients.

Another area of interest is the use of regenerative medicine techniques, such as stem cell therapy. Stem cells have the potential to differentiate into various cell types and promote healing and regeneration in damaged tissues. Researchers are exploring the use of stem cells to repair and regenerate tissues affected by fibromyalgia, potentially offering a new avenue for treatment. Although still in the early stages of research, stem cell therapy holds promise for the future of fibromyalgia treatment.

Ongoing Research

Current research into fibromyalgia is focused on understanding the underlying mechanisms of the condition and identifying biomarkers that can aid in diagnosis and treatment. One area of study involves investigating the role of central sensitization, a condition in which the central nervous system becomes hypersensitive to stimuli, leading to increased pain perception. Researchers are exploring the genetic and molecular factors that contribute to central sensitization in fibromyalgia, aiming to develop targeted therapies that can modulate these pathways and reduce pain.

Another focus of research is the role of the immune system and inflammation in fibromyalgia. Studies are examining the interactions between the nervous system and the immune system, investigating how inflammatory processes contribute to pain and other symptoms. Identifying specific inflammatory markers associated with fibromyalgia could lead to the development of new anti-inflammatory treatments that target these pathways.

Advances in neuroimaging technology are also enhancing our understanding of fibromyalgia. Functional magnetic resonance imaging (fMRI) and positron emission tomography (PET) scans are being used to study brain activity and connectivity in fibromyalgia patients. These imaging techniques allow researchers to visualize changes in brain regions involved in pain processing, emotional regulation, and cognitive function. By identifying distinct patterns of brain activity associated with fibromyalgia, researchers hope to develop more accurate diagnostic tools and personalized treatment approaches.

Genetic research is another promising area of study. Scientists are investigating the genetic variations that may predispose individuals to fibromyalgia. By identifying specific genes and genetic markers associated with the condition, researchers aim to develop genetic tests that can aid in diagnosis and provide insights into personalized treatment strategies. Understanding the genetic basis of fibromyalgia could also lead to the development of targeted therapies that address the underlying genetic factors contributing to the condition.

Clinical trials continue to play a crucial role in advancing fibromyalgia treatment. Researchers are conducting trials to test the safety and efficacy of new medications, therapies, and interventions. These trials provide valuable data on the potential benefits and risks of emerging treatments, helping to identify effective options for managing fibromyalgia. Participation in clinical trials offers patients the opportunity to access cutting-edge treatments and contribute to the advancement of fibromyalgia research.

Growing Awareness and Advocacy

The future of fibromyalgia is also being shaped by growing awareness and advocacy efforts. Increased public awareness of fibromyalgia is leading to greater recognition of the condition and its impact on individuals' lives. Advocacy organizations, such as the National Fibromyalgia Association (NFA) and the Fibromyalgia Network, are working tirelessly to raise awareness, provide education, and advocate for research funding and policy changes. These organizations offer resources, support, and community for individuals living with fibromyalgia and their families.

Efforts to improve education and training for healthcare providers are also underway. Enhancing healthcare providers' understanding of fibromyalgia can lead to earlier diagnosis, more effective treatment, and better patient outcomes. Medical schools and continuing education programs are incorporating fibromyalgia education into their curricula, ensuring that future healthcare professionals are equipped with the knowledge and skills to manage the condition effectively.

CONCLUSION

Living with fibromyalgia is undoubtedly a journey filled with challenges, but it is also one that can be navigated with knowledge, support, and proactive management. Fibromyalgia: Understanding Symptoms, Treatments, and Self-Help Strategies has aimed to provide you with a comprehensive resource to better understand this complex condition and to equip you with the tools and strategies necessary for effective management.

Throughout this book, we have explored the multifaceted nature of fibromyalgia, starting with its history and fundamental understanding in Chapter 1: Fibromyalgia 101. We delved into the wide array of symptoms that characterize fibromyalgia in Chapter 2: The Signs & Symptoms, helping you recognize and address the diverse manifestations of this condition.

Chapter 3: Getting Diagnosed provided insights into the often complicated diagnostic process, highlighting the importance of accurate diagnosis and the professionals who can assist you. Understanding the various treatment options available is crucial, and Chapter 4: Treating Fibromyalgia with Medication and Chapter 5: Additional Treatment Options offered a thorough overview of both conventional and alternative therapies.

We recognized that self-help strategies are a cornerstone of managing fibromyalgia. Chapter 6: Self-Help Techniques provided practical advice on diet, sleep, exercise, stress management, and symptom tracking, empowering you to take control of your health. Similarly, Chapter 7: Supplements and Herbal Remedies explored natural therapies that can complement your treatment plan.

Living well with fibromyalgia requires a holistic approach that considers all aspects of life. Chapter 8: Living with Fibromyalgia discussed strategies for balancing work, school, home life, and social interactions, ensuring you can maintain a good quality of life despite the challenges posed by fibromyalgia.

Finally, Chapter 9: The Future of Fibromyalgia looked ahead to the promising advancements in research and treatment. With emerging therapies, ongoing studies, and increased awareness, there is hope for more effective management and improved outcomes for those living with fibromyalgia.

As you continue your journey with fibromyalgia, remember that you are not alone. Building a strong support network, staying informed about new developments, and advocating for your needs are essential steps in managing this condition. Knowledge is power, and by understanding fibromyalgia and exploring various treatment and self-help strategies, you can make informed decisions that positively impact your health and well-being.

While fibromyalgia presents significant challenges, it also offers an opportunity to develop resilience, adaptability, and a deeper understanding of your own body. Embrace the tools and strategies discussed in this book, and tailor them to your unique needs. Be patient with yourself, celebrate your progress, and seek support when needed.

This book is intended to be a guide and a source of support for anyone affected by fibromyalgia. Whether you are newly diagnosed, have been living with the condition for years, or are supporting a loved one, the information and insights provided here are meant to empower you to live a fulfilling and balanced life.

Thank you for embarking on this journey with me. I hope that this book has provided you with valuable knowledge and practical tools to navigate the complexities of fibromyalgia. Remember, the path to managing fibromyalgia is a personal one, and you have the strength and resources to find your way.

Printed in Great Britain
by Amazon